W0259767

Praise for *The Nervous System Workbook*

"Deb Dana's wonderful workbook guides you step-by-step through learning about your nervous system and how to bring it back into balance when life is challenging. The tools and practices in this workbook are gifts you can give yourself over and over again."

Diane Poole Heller, PhD
author of *The Power of Attachment*

"Deb Dana masterfully demystifies the complexities of the Polyvagal Theory, offering readers an empowering journey towards self-regulation. Each exercise serves as a road map towards greater resilience and emotional balance, paving the way for optimal well-being. *The Nervous System Workbook* is a must-read for anyone seeking to harness the power of their nervous system for a more fulfilling life."

Stephen W. Porges, PhD
creator of the Polyvagal Theory

"Deb Dana's *Nervous System Workbook* speaks in a beautifully compassionate, non-pathologizing voice directly to the individual using it. The steps toward befriending and tending the nervous system are spelled out in simple exercises that build on each other. The calming sense of ease in this approach can be felt on every page."

Janina Fisher
author of *Healing the Fragmented Selves of Trauma Survivors*

"Weaving together insights from contemporary neuroscience and years of clinical practice, this workbook offers clear, step-by-step, engaging exercises that can help anyone better understand their nervous system and move from stress and fear toward stability, equanimity, and harmony. With warmth, humor, and a wise understanding of our differences, Deb Dana gives us a banquet of approaches so that we all can find our way to live a calmer, richer, more deeply connected and rewarding life."

Ronald D. Siegel, PsyD

Harvard Medical School, author of

The Extraordinary Gift of Being Ordinary

"*The Nervous System Workbook* by Deb Dana beautifully illustrates how to tend and befriend your nervous system! It translates the science of connection into easy, clear, and digestible tools and practices to help you find a sense of safety in your body and connection with others. It's a must-read for everyone who knows or wants to know 'home' in themselves and in the world."

Pat Ogden, PhD

founder and CEO of Sensorimotor Psychotherapy Institute

the nervous system workbook

Also by Deb Dana

Anchored: How to Befriend Your Nervous System Using Polyvagal Theory

Befriending Your Nervous System: Looking through the Lens of Polyvagal Theory (audio program)

Polyvagal Card Deck

Polyvagal Exercises for Safety and Connection: 50 Client-Centered Practices

Polyvagal Flip Chart

Polyvagal Practices: Anchoring the Self in Safety

Polyvagal Prompts: Finding Connection and Joy Through Guided Explorations (with Courtney Rolfe)

The Polyvagal Theory in Therapy: Engaging the Rhythm of Regulation

the nervous system workbook

practical exercises to ease anxiety, find safety and come home to yourself using polyvagal theory

DEB DANA

Vermilion
LONDON

1

Vermilion, an imprint of Ebury Publishing
One Embassy Gardens, 8 Viaduct Gardens,
Nine Elms, London SW11 7BW

Vermilion is part of the Penguin Random House group of companies
whose addresses can be found at global.penguinrandomhouse.com

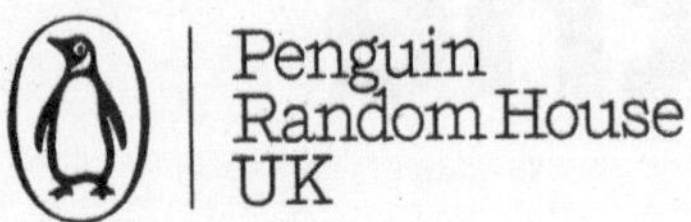

Copyright © Deborah A. Dana 2024

Deborah A. Dana has asserted her right to be identified as the author of this Work in accordance with the Copyright, Designs and Patents Act 1988

No part of this book may be used or reproduced in any manner for the purpose of training artificial intelligence technologies or systems. In accordance with Article 4(3) of the DSM Directive 2019/790, Penguin Random House expressly reserves this work from the text and data mining exception.

First published in Great Britain by Vermilion in 2024
First published in the United States of America by Sounds True in 2024

www.penguin.co.uk

A CIP catalogue record for this book is available from the British Library

ISBN 9781785045714

Printed and bound in Great Britain by Clays Ltd, Elcograf S.p.A.

The authorised representative in the EEA is Penguin Random House Ireland, Morrison Chambers, 32 Nassau Street, Dublin D02 YH68

Penguin Random House is committed to a sustainable future for our business, our readers and our planet. This book is made from Forest Stewardship Council® certified paper.

The information in this book has been compiled as general guidance on the specific subjects addressed. It is not a substitute and not to be relied on for medical, healthcare or pharmaceutical professional advice. Please consult your GP before changing, stopping or starting any medical treatment. So far as the author is aware the information given is correct and up to date as at September 2024. Practice, laws and regulations all change and the reader should obtain up to date professional advice on any such issues. The authors and publishers disclaim, as far as the law allows, any liability arising directly or indirectly from the use, or misuse, of the information contained in this book.

contents

introduction

While you may think your brain directs your daily experiences, in fact the way you move through the world—the stories about who you are, how the world works, what you do, and how you feel—begins in your body with the autonomic nervous system. Your nervous system shapes your experiences of safety and connection and guides the way you navigate living, loving, and working. Yet, up until now, most of us have not been taught what the nervous system does or how it works. Without a basic understanding of this essential system, you're in the dark and missing opportunities to experience your days differently and live your life with greater ease. To get to know your nervous system, you need to become familiar with Polyvagal Theory. Developed by renowned scientist Dr. Stephen Porges, Polyvagal Theory explains the science of safety and connection and gives you a map of your nervous system to guide your exploration. This theory is the foundation of this workbook.

My passion, and the intention of this workbook, is translating the science of connection—what I like to call the science of feeling safe enough to fall in love with life—into a language that is easy to understand and developing tools and practices to help you partner with your nervous system and bring more moments of regulation and connection into your daily life. As a clinician and author specializing in using the lens of Polyvagal Theory to understand and resolve the impact of trauma in our lives and create ways of being that honor the role of the autonomic nervous system, I am excited to be your guide in this exploration of your nervous system.

For ten years I have collaborated with Dr. Porges as a mentor, coauthor, colleague, and friend to bring Polyvagal Theory into clinical application. Lately, I have expanded my work to bring Polyvagal Theory to communities outside the clinical arena so everyone can experience the many benefits of a regulated nervous system and navigate life with greater ease. What I love about the nervous system is that it is the common denominator in our human experience. We all have a nervous system that works in similar ways and, in a world that often feels disconnected, that shared experience brings us together. When I look at myself and others through the lens of the nervous system, I recognize that we are all trying to find the state of safety that supports connection.

A regulated nervous system is fundamental to the process of navigating the world with a sense of safety and ease. Healing happens as we increase our capacity for regulation.

While I have been exploring this work for many years and have wisdom and expertise to share, I also have times when I'm challenged to hold onto regulation and find myself in moments of messiness. As you work through the exercises in this workbook, remember that we all start from the same place—a place of seeking safety and connection. We're all human and we're all on this journey together.

Each one of us encounters problems over the course of a day. Some are more easily managed than others, but no matter where an experience lands on the continuum of mild to traumatic, understanding how the nervous system works is the path to finding the way back to regulation. When the inner workings of our biology are a mystery to us, we feel as if we're at the mercy of unknown, unexplainable, and unpredictable experiences. Naturally this results in feelings of anxiety and distress, feelings familiar to many of us. But the beauty is that once you know how your nervous system works, you can work *with* it. You can track your journey out of dysregulation with a roadmap to find your way back to safety.

> **With a basic understanding of the ways the nervous system works, you can partner with your nervous system and begin to make sense of why you think and act in the ways you do. You can more easily navigate the ordinary, and sometimes extraordinary, experiences of daily living.**

The Nervous System Workbook introduces you to your nervous system and shows you how to partner with it to bring a bit more safety, connection, and even joy to your life. You'll add new words to your vocabulary and explore some basic concepts, but you don't have to become a scientist. Befriending your nervous system is a gentle process of discovery and learning. Curiosity and a willingness to explore are all you need.

How the Nervous System Works

The autonomic nervous system could also be called the *automatic* nervous system since it takes care of your body's basic housekeeping responsibilities, things that the body does seemingly effortlessly (e.g., breath, heart rate, digestion), without needing to pay attention to them. Imagine having to remind your heart to beat, your lungs to breathe, or your digestive system to do its job. All your attention would be focused on these basic life functions leaving no room for thinking about anything else. Instead, we can feel grateful that, despite our lack of awareness, we have this innate system that keeps everything working.

Maybe your nervous system has done a pretty good job so far so you're wondering why you need to learn more about it. Like many things in our lives, when we really start to understand how something works, and how it benefits us, we discover a new way of relating to it. As we take the mystery out of the way the nervous system works and begin to get to know it, we recognize the power of autonomic awareness in daily life to bring kindness, self-compassion, ease, and even joy. Increased understanding presents us with new and hopeful opportunities, such as moving from irritation or frustration with what our nervous system is doing to having compassion and appreciation for its design.

It's a normal human experience to move through autonomic states in both small shifts and bigger ways many times a day. Consider the states you have already experienced today in moments of ease, small slightly charged moments, others that felt empty, or even more intense moments of fight, flight, or collapse. The common experience of moving in and out of states is not itself a barrier to well-being. It's only when you move out of safety and connection into a survival response and can't find your way back to a state of regulation that you suffer physically and psychologically. It's normal and expected to not feel regulated 24 hours a day and instead move in and out of different states. What you'll focus on in this workbook is how to become aware of where you are and *how to return to regulation*. Coming back to safety, learning to come home to yourself every day, is the skill this book offers.

As you notice what your nervous system is doing, you naturally become curious about what it is reacting to and trying to tell you about what it needs. When you learn to listen and speak the language of the nervous system, you can respond to what's happening in the moment in more intentional ways, ways that lead to safety and connection. I call this getting-to-know process "befriending your nervous system." Many of us are unaware of the important information being sent from our bodies to our brains through autonomic pathways. When you partner with your nervous system, rather than ignoring it, you can tune in and begin to nurture its well-being.

One way to think about the job of the nervous system is that it is always working on your behalf in service of your safety.

It detects changes in your internal environment and monitors the safety of your external environment, regulates your heartbeat and breathing rate, and matches your energy level to the needs of the moment. In addition to managing your physical needs, the nervous system is also the place where your stories about yourself and the world begin. Unlike the saying "what happens in Vegas stays in Vegas," what happens in the nervous system does not stay in the nervous system. Instead, information about events occurring in the nervous system travel from the body's organs to the brain along an autonomic pathway. When the information arrives in the brain, the brain creates a story to make sense of what it's hearing and learning. I don't know about you, but my brain can make up some incredible and incredulous stories!

The wonderful thing about this system is that it can change. You have the power to shape new patterns, which is some of the work you'll be doing in this workbook. The three principles below provide us with a roadmap for how the nervous system works.

Organizing Principles

1. **Autonomic Hierarchy:** The three building blocks that work in sequence and come with preset pathways
2. **Neuroception:** The built-in surveillance system that is always watching for signs of safety and warns about danger ahead
3. **Co-regulation:** The way to safely connect with others, a necessary ingredient for well-being

Autonomic Hierarchy: The Building Blocks of Experience

Through the process of evolution, the three building blocks of the nervous system came into being one after the other: dorsal vagal around 500 million years ago, sympathetic around 400 million years ago, and ventral vagal around 200 million years ago. As each new system emerged, it joined the older system rather than replacing it. This sequential order, called the autonomic hierarchy, is key to understanding how the nervous system anchors in regulation and reacts to challenges in daily living. Each of these building blocks works in a specific way, affecting your biology through connections inside the body and impacting your psychology by directing how you see, sense, and engage with the world around you.

Ventral Vagal

The ventral vagal building block, the newest of the three, provides a pathway to health and well-being and the place where life feels manageable. This building block allows you to connect and communicate with others, join groups, and be happy on your own. The common irritations of daily living don't feel so big and when your coffee spills or the commute is too slow, instead of getting angry or anxious, you're able to "go with the flow." To get a feel for this system, remember sitting and talking with a friend, think about walking in nature feeling connected to the earth, or, if you have a dog or cat, imagine them curled up beside you.

Sympathetic

Following the pattern of the hierarchy, when something happens that feels overwhelming, when too many things happen all at once, or when it seems like life is a series of never-ending challenges, you move down a step to the next building block, the action-taking sympathetic pathway. This is commonly known as the place of fight-and-flight. When your to-do list doesn't ever seem to get smaller, when there is never quite enough money to make ends meet, or when it feels like your partner is always distracted, you lose your sense of being safe in the present moment and being able to see a larger picture and you react either by attacking or escaping. To get a flavor of the mobilization of this system imagine a shark attacking or a fish darting to escape.

Dorsal Vagal

If you continue to feel trapped in a cycle of endless challenges with no way out and no way to manage, you follow the hierarchy down the final step to the first building block of the nervous system: the dorsal vagal feeling of collapse, shutdown, and disconnection. Here, the spilled coffee, the never-ending to-do list, and the partner who never seems to be present no longer matter. You begin to shut down and disconnect. You may still go through the motions but with no energy to care. You lose hope that anything will ever change. To get a sense of this part of the system, think about a turtle moving slowly and steadily through the world. When scared, the turtle immobilizes, disappears into its shell, and waits until it feels safe enough to peek out at the world again.

Moving Between States

We naturally travel between states, routinely moving out of ventral regulation into sympathetic or dorsal dysregulation and back again. Leaving regulation isn't the problem. In fact, the goal is not to stay in a state of regulation but rather to know where you are, recognize when you're moving out of regulation and being pulled into a survival response, and be able to return to regulation. The ability to flexibly move between states is a sign of well-being and resilience. It is when you are caught in dysregulation, unable to find your way back to regulation, that you feel distress. When you get pulled out of ventral safety and connection and get lost in a place of dysregulation, you move from flexibility to rigidity and feel the effects of a nervous system that is stuck in the intensity of sympathetic mobilization or dorsal shutdown.

When anchored in the regulating energy of the ventral vagal state, the autonomic nervous system is in balance, and you experience the sense of well-being that comes with a feeling of healthy homeostasis. In times of challenge, you can reflect (rather than react), collaborate, and communicate. Stop for a moment and think about a time when you felt regulated and solved a problem on your own or found a solution with someone else. If you're not successful in meeting and managing a challenge, you move out of regulation into sympathetic mobilization and the energy of fight-and-flight. Pause here and remember a time when you experienced that intensely activating energy and were driven to stay and argue or felt desperate to get away. Finally, if taking action doesn't resolve the challenge and you feel trapped, you move to dorsal vagal shutdown. Think about a time when you felt like giving up or going along without really being present or caring. And now, because of the way the nervous system was formed, one building block on top of another, to return to safety and regulation from the state of collapse, you need to travel through sympathetic mobilization without getting caught in a fight-and-flight response. A moment of safe mobilization can take many forms. It might start with a small body movement, a shared look with someone, or even a thought that feels like the beginning of a possibility. The essential element of this moment of mobilization is a return of energy that is not so big or intense that it becomes a cue of danger but rather is felt as a cue of safety that shows the way back to regulation. From this safe starting point, you can continue to feel energy returning and find your way back to ventral regulation.

Neuroception: Your Internal Surveillance System

The second principle of Polyvagal Theory, the internal surveillance system, is defined by the wonderfully descriptive word *neuroception*. Stephen Porges created this word to illustrate how the nervous system (*neuro*) is aware of (*ception*) signs of safety and signals of danger.

With a neuroception of safety, you move out into the world and into connection. A neuroception of danger brings a move into sympathetic fight-and-flight, while a neuroception of intense danger takes you into dorsal vagal collapse and shutdown.

Neuroception follows three streams of awareness: inside, outside, and between. **Inside listening** happens as neuroception attends to what's going on inside your body—to your heartbeat, breath rhythms, and muscle action—and inside your organs, especially those involved with your digestion. **Outside listening** begins in your immediate environment (where you are physically located) and then expands out into the larger world to include neighborhoods, nations, and the global community. The third stream of awareness, **listening between**, is the way your nervous system communicates with other systems one-on-one or with a group of people. These three streams of embodied listening are always working, micro-moment to micro-moment, below the level of your conscious awareness. Running in the background, neuroception brings the autonomic state changes that either invite you into connection with people, places, and experiences or move you away from connection into the protection of fight, flight, or shutdown.

Your stories, and how you think, feel, and act, begin with neuroception. And while you can't work directly with neuroception, you can work with your body's response to it. When you bring perception to neuroception, you bring an otherwise unconscious experience into awareness. You can work with your experience by taking the implicit experience of neuroception, explicitly noticing it, and turning your attention toward the state that has come alive. As you keep traveling the pathway of awareness, you connect with feelings, beliefs, behaviors, and finally the story that takes you through your days. When you learn to attend to neuroception, you can begin to shape your story in new ways.

Co-regulation: Wired for Connection

In our evolutionary history, being a part of a group was essential for survival. There was strength in numbers. This leads us to the third principle of Polyvagal Theory—the need for finding safe connection with others in experiences of co-regulation. Co-regulation, regulating with another, is necessary for surviving and thriving. You come into the world unable to fend for yourself and, for the first years of life, you need to be cared for by others. You are physically unable to regulate on your own and naturally turn toward the people around you to meet both physical and emotional survival needs. As you grow, these experiences of co-regulation offer a foundation to explore regulating on your own.

Even as you learn to self-regulate, the need for co-regulation continues. This is both an essential ingredient for well-being and a challenge to negotiate. In order to co-regulate, I have to feel safe with you, you have to feel safe with me, and we have to find a way to come into connection and regulate with each other. You turn to a friend to listen or look to a family member for help. You depend on certain people in your life to show up with a regulated system when you're in need. And although many of us may not have predictably safe, regulated people to connect with, and co-regulation isn't always possible, it is important to recognize that we have a built-in biological need for one another. While the world seems to be increasingly focused on self-regulation and independence, co-regulation is the foundation for safely navigating daily living.

We carry the ongoing need to connect with others and every day we long for, and look for, opportunities to co-regulate.

It is through these three principles—hierarchy, neuroception, and co-regulation—that you have both a way to acknowledge the role that biology has in shaping how you move through the world and a guide to engaging with your biology in ways that bring about well-being.

How to Use This Workbook

What happens when someone tells you what you should do and goes on to tell you how you should do it? Rather than feeling cared about, many of us feel pressured. How about if someone asks you what appeals to you or offers you a range of options and lets you choose? When that happens most of us feel like the other person is interested in our feelings and cares about what we want. In general, we respond to a warm invitation with curiosity and have a negative reaction to a demand.

This workbook is a warm invitation to you, and I hope you meet it with curiosity and openness. If you feel you have to work from cover to cover, if you push yourself to complete one page every day or go through the workbook never looking ahead or skipping around, you will likely feel frustrated and may end up giving up. Even if you force yourself to do all the exercises, when you reach the end you'll probably wonder why you bothered. While the goal *is* to complete all the exercises, the pathway to success isn't a straight line. Proceed with an attitude of curiosity and go where you feel pulled on any given day. Follow your nervous system as you work through these exercises. When you open the workbook, ask yourself what will feel nourishing in this moment and choose the exercise that fits. There's no rush; take as much time as you want as you work toward completing all the exercises.

The workbook is designed in two parts: part 1: Befriending Your Nervous System and part 2: Coming Home to Safety and Connection. Part 1 offers a variety of pathways to get to know how your nervous system works. There are exercises that use language, imagery, movement, and body awareness, giving you lots of ways to practice befriending. Part 1 helps you discover how your nervous system works and how to work with it. Part 2 builds on that foundation by taking you into the world of autonomic patterns with exercises that are designed to help you reach for regulation in challenging moments and help you reshape your system in the direction of connection. Remember, even though the process is to complete the exercises in part 1 and then move on to part 2, there is no specific order within each part that you need to follow. Listen to your nervous system and let it guide your choice.

I'm often asked about the impact of neurodiversity when working with the nervous system. When it comes to thinking about the ways we are wired, the starting point for everyone, whether you identify as neurodiverse or neurotypical, is to get to know your nervous system. The same is true if you have health challenges or other conditions that impact your nervous system. Everyone's nervous system is organized around the three principles of hierarchy, neuroception, and co-regulation and we each travel along a personal continuum of response. No two nervous systems are exactly alike and getting to know how your nervous system works leads you along the path to becoming an active operator of your own system no matter how it is wired.

A regulated nervous system is fundamental to navigating the world with a sense of safety and ease.

When you learn to befriend the nervous system and anchor in autonomic safety, you'll move through the world in a new way and experience the powerful benefits that come with finding your personal pathways to calm and connection.

As you get ready to turn the page and begin your journey of exploration, remember: there is no right way or wrong way . . . there is only the way of your nervous system!

part one

befriending your nervous system

Think about a close friend and recall how that relationship began and grew. You probably didn't just meet and in that moment your friendship was fully formed. Becoming friends, or befriending, takes time and attention. Each time you meet you get to know each other a bit more. You build trust over time. You learn about each other's habits, discover how to talk to each other, and because the relationship makes you happy, you find ways to stay in connection. Befriending your nervous system is a similar process. When you're introduced to your nervous system, you learn just a bit about its inner workings at first. The key is to stay curious about how it works *and* how you work with it. Eventually you'll learn how to work together in the process of befriending.

Friendship requires trust, communication, time spent in connection, care, compassion, and curiosity. It is possible to create that with your nervous system. The exercises in this section are designed to help you partner with your nervous system and build those qualities. When you befriend your nervous system the inevitable challenges you face as you go through your days aren't quite so formidable and you find you can navigate life more easily.

→ **The process of befriending is an ongoing journey of discovery. Let's begin.**

my system in balance

Have you ever experienced a moment when you felt like you were in a flow? Have you had a day when things were easy and you felt okay? It is your nervous system that shapes these experiences. When your nervous system is regulated, you come into balance with a sense of stability, equanimity, and harmony.

Your ventral system, the system of safety and connection, makes these positive feelings possible. When ventral is leading the way, the survival energy of fight-and-flight shifts into energy that is alive, active, and supportive to you as you move through your day. Shutting down is no longer needed as a survival strategy and instead, your dorsal system now lends its support by regulating your digestion in healthy ways, delivering nutrients to nourish you. As you get to know your system you will learn to recognize those nourishing moments and lean into them. You'll discover that it's possible to be in balance.

This exercise is a way to visualize your system in balance through color, so you'll want to have markers or crayons handy to do this. The center circle represents dorsal, the middle circle represents sympathetic, and the outer circle represents ventral.

Let's begin in the center with your dorsal circle.

The energy here is slow and steady, bringing a sense of being grounded. Color in the center circle with colors that illustrate this experience for you. Don't overthink it; just let your intuition guide you.

Next, choose colors to illustrate the middle circle representing your sympathetic system and color it in.

Here the energy is active and alive, moving you through the day.

Now let's move on to the outer ventral circle.

There is a flow to the energy here. This is the place that anchors you in regulation and connection and holds the other two states in a circle of safety. Color it in with colors that illustrate this experience.

When you've colored in all your circles, look at the palettes for each circle and then see how the shades come together, creating a picture of balance.

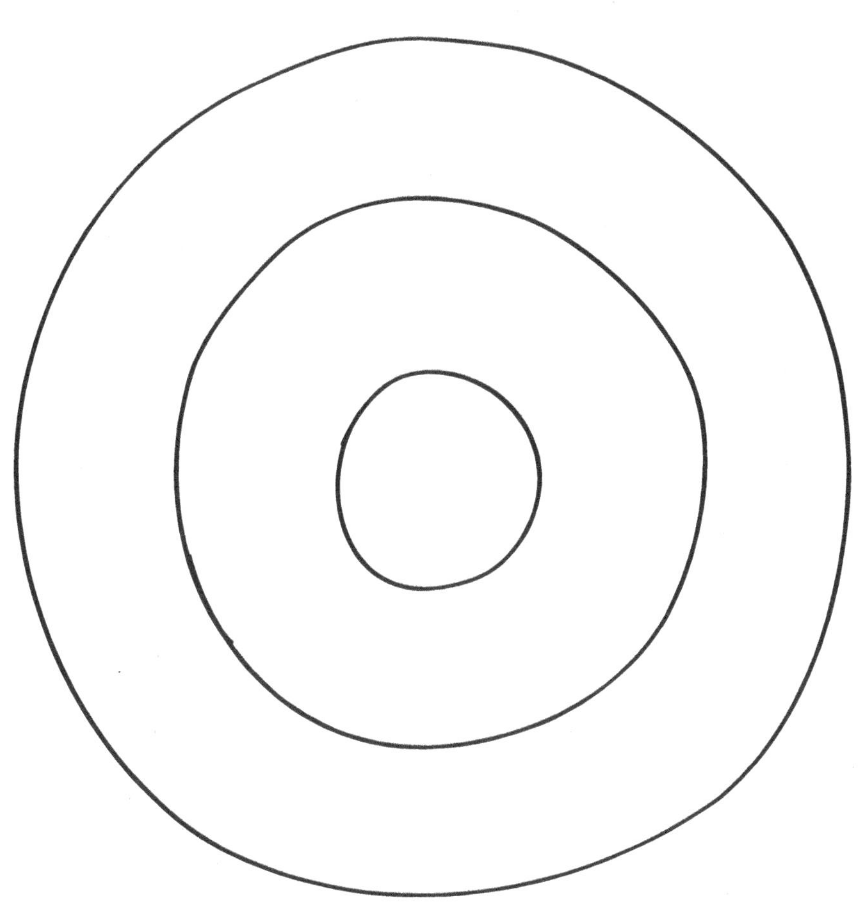

Finally, take a moment to reflect on what it's like to see your system in balance in this way and, moving beyond this exercise, envision for a moment feeling in balance.

How do you experience *being* in balance?

For more on envisioning your system in balance, listen to this Three Circles Visualization audio practice soundstrue.com/the-nervous-system-workbook-bonus.

anchored in safety

Physical and emotional health and well-being are possible when your nervous system is anchored in regulation. When this happens, the common irritations of daily living don't feel so big, life becomes more manageable, and the world feels alive with possibilities. Sometimes these moments are fleeting and sometimes they are longer lasting. When you think about the past week, was there a moment, or even a micro-moment, when you felt a sense of regulation?

This exercise helps you get to know what happens when you are in a state of regulation so you can recognize the signs. You'll learn to identify what happens in your body, what you think, how you feel, and what your behaviors are. Recognizing is the first step in inviting more moments of regulation into your life.

Begin in the center of the illustration by drawing a shape that represents your feeling of being anchored in safety.

I often choose a heart, but you choose a shape that feels right for you. Now label your shape with a word(s) that defines this experience for you. I like the words *safe* and *connected*. What word(s) helps you feel anchored in safety?

Last, fill in the circles with words that represent how you feel in your body sensations, behaviors, emotions, and thoughts when you are anchored in safety.

What happens in each of these categories when you feel safe and okay? Write your words for each inside the corresponding circle.

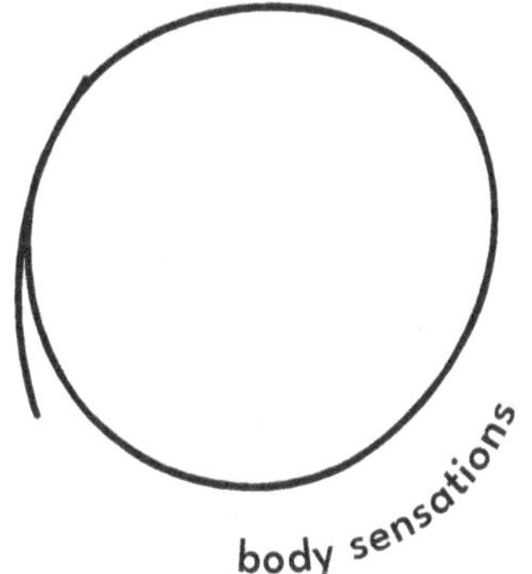
body sensations

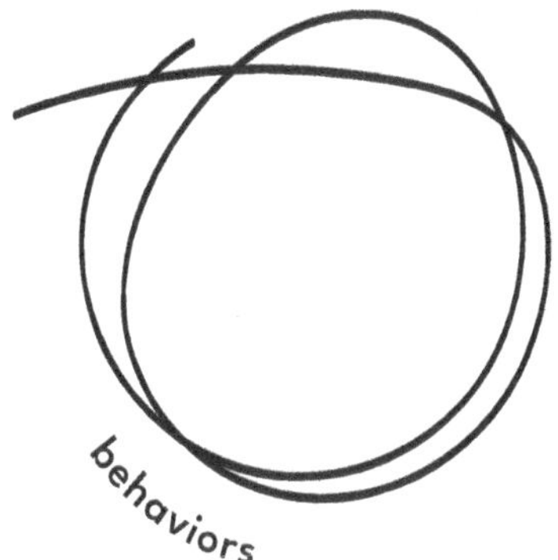
behaviors

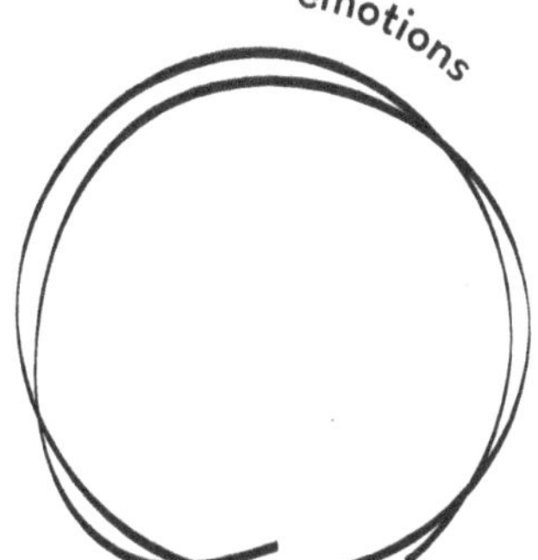
emotions

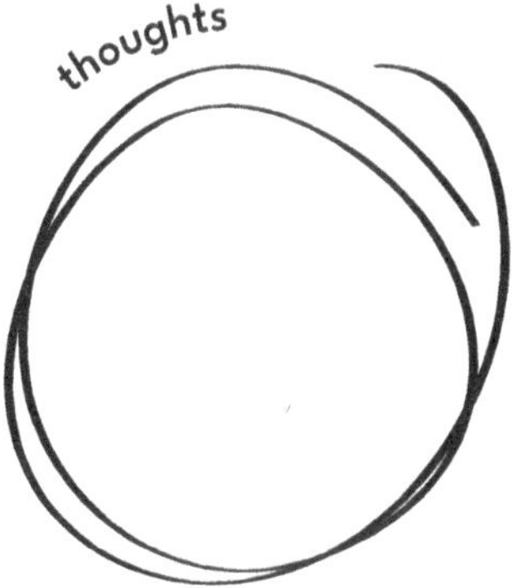
thoughts

in service of survival

The motto of the nervous system is *in service of safety.* When daily life feels overwhelming, your nervous system reacts to support and protect you. This exercise uses the same structure as in "Anchored in Safety" and continues the befriending process by helping you identify the ways in which your two survival states activate. Knowing how your body, behaviors, feelings, and thoughts work when you're in a survival state gives you the information you need to recognize when you move into dysregulation.

Part 1

When you lose your sense of feeling safe, the first place you go is into fight-and-flight. When a moment feels overwhelming, when too many things happen all at once, or when it seems like life is a series of never-ending challenges that you can't ever meet, you are pushed into dysregulation, which is experienced as some aspect of anger and anxiety.

Begin in the center of the illustration space and draw a shape that represents your fight-and-flight system.

I like a shape with angles and edges and often draw a lightning bolt. Take time to choose the shape that feels personal to you. Now label your shape with a word(s) that defines this experience for you. My words are chaotic and scary. What words describe dysregulation for you?

Next, move to the circles for body sensations, behaviors, emotions, and thoughts. What happens in each of these categories when you feel unsafe, angry, or anxious? Write your words for each inside the corresponding circle.

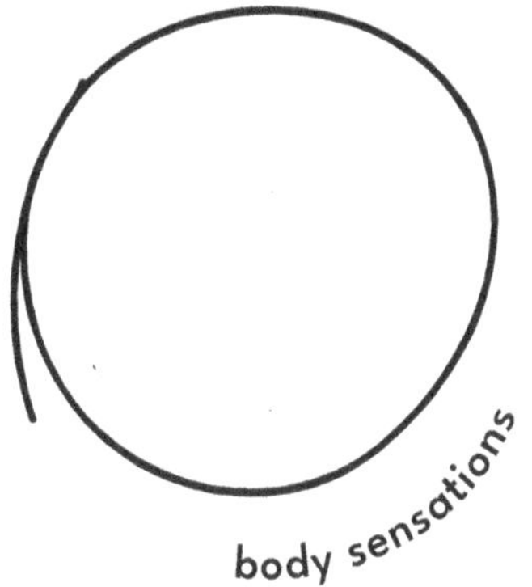
body sensations

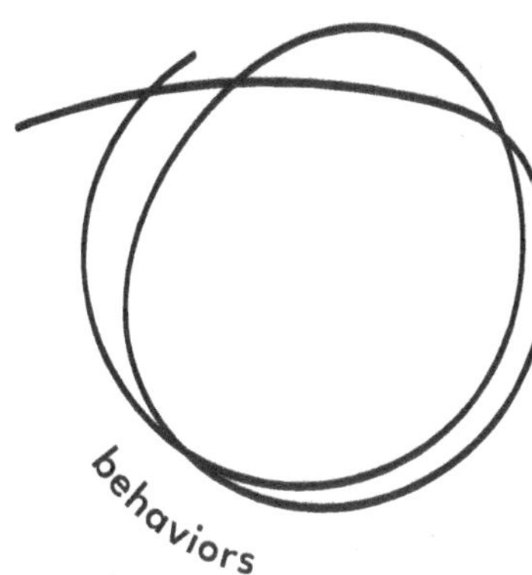
behaviors

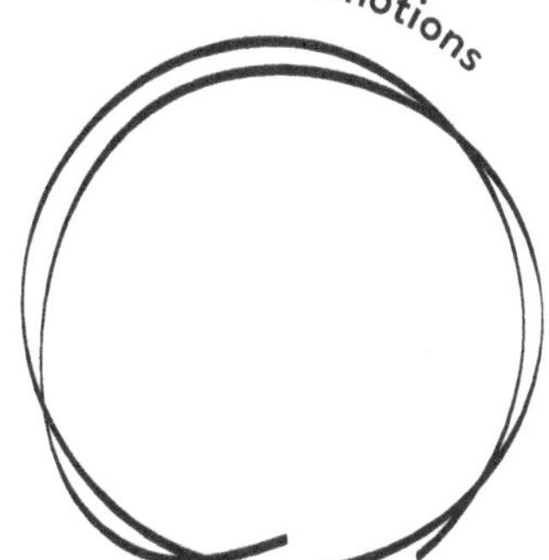
emotions

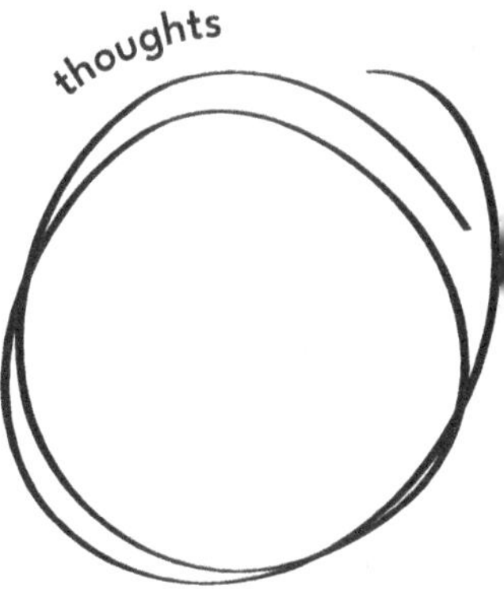
thoughts

Part 2

Shutting down is a natural response to feeling trapped in a cycle of endless challenges with no way out and no way to manage. Life feels that way sometimes and it can seem like the only option is to shut down, go numb, opt out. As the energy drains from your body, you are pulled into collapse and begin to lose hope that anything will ever get better. This normal—albeit dysregulated—response is your nervous system attempting to help you escape the overwhelming challenges you are faced with.

In the center of the illustration space, draw a shape that represents your system of collapse and shutdown.

To me this feels like a dead place and I often just draw a flat line. Take time to choose the shape that is meaningful to you. Label your shape with a word(s) that defines this experience for you. My words are *lost* and *invisible.*

Next, write words in the circles for body sensations, behaviors, emotions, and thoughts that describe when you feel shut down, drained of energy, and unable to connect. What happens in each of these categories?

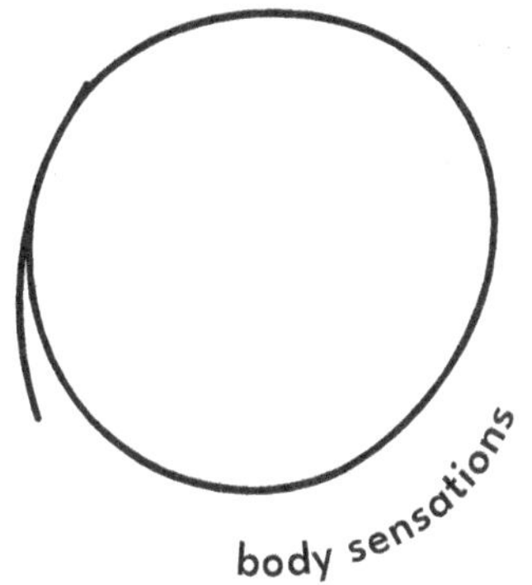
body sensations

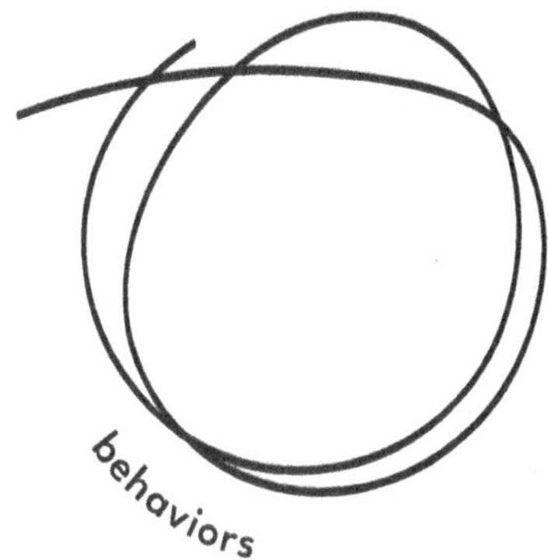
behaviors

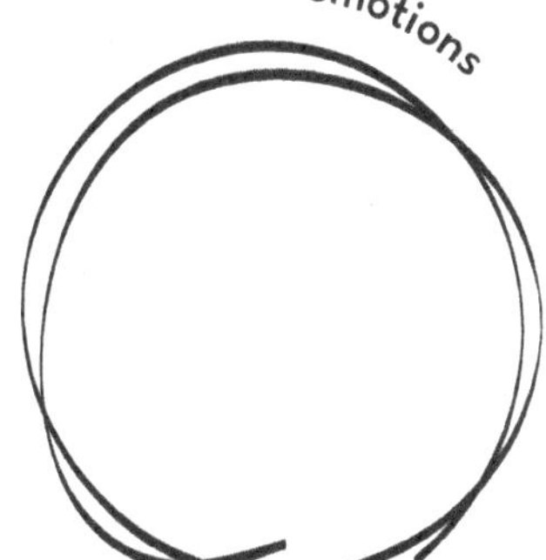
emotions

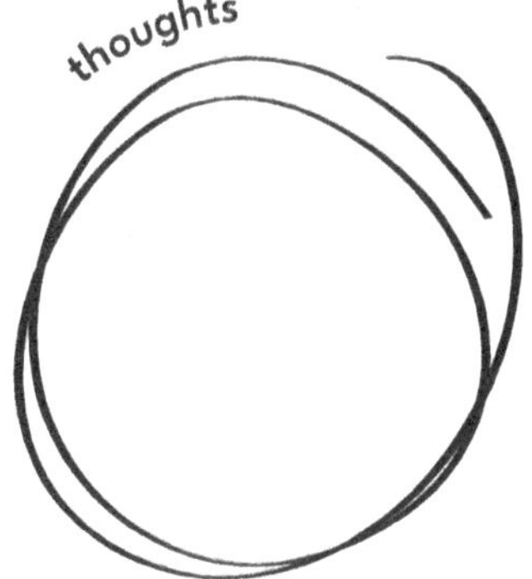
thoughts

predictable pathways

Your nervous system is built to keep you safe and help you survive moments of danger. To do this, it uses the energy of regulation and balance and survival strategies of fight-and-flight, collapse, and shutdown. All of these are your body's way of helping you. Over the course of a day, you regularly move in and out of regulation. Feeling small moments of distress and quickly returning to regulation is a normal part of daily life and is actually a good thing because it builds resilience. Over time you learn that you can take steps to return to regulation.

The wonderful thing about the nervous system is that it is predictable. This means when you feel overwhelmed you can reliably count on moving out of regulation and into anxiety and anger. I've been known to rant to a friend, stomp around the house, or just get up and leave.

What do you do when you feel overwhelmed?

Sometimes my ranting and stomping helps me release some of my energy and I find the way back to regulation.

Has that happened for you? What works to help you release some energy and come back to regulation?

Other times, instead of returning to regulation, you get pulled deeper into dysregulation and shutdown. When I land here, I just go through the motions without the energy to care. Sometimes I stay in my pajamas and sit on the couch all day.

What happens for you?

What can you call on to return to regulation from here? To move out of shutdown you need just a bit of energy to return to start you on the path back to regulation. Think about the little things that help you begin to feel less shut down. I find making small movements, texting with someone, or listening to music helps.

What works to help you feel some energy returning and find your way back to regulation?

at home in regulation

Your nervous system comes with built-in pathways of safety and connection. When you travel those pathways and arrive in a state of regulation you have found your way home. Is this a place that's familiar to you or is this a place you don't know well? Maybe you remember this home in regulation but recently you've been struggling to find your way. With images and imagination, you can create the landscape of your regulated system with the elements and details that bring a sense of safety and connection alive. You can use this landscape when you need to find your way home to regulation and re-experience what it's like to inhabit that nourishing place. You can call on this place and the feelings it brings in times of distress.

Imagine you have entered the landscape of regulation—a place inside yourself where you feel safe, comfortable, and happy.

What do you see as you look around? Are there elements of the natural world? A house, animals, people? What are the colors and energy here? What do you smell? What do you hear? Is there a path to walk or a place to rest? Take time to explore.

Use this space to write about, or illustrate, your home in regulation.

my home away from home

When you're in need of protection, your nervous system comes to your rescue. It has the option of two different survival states, each with its own strategy. One initiates an active response to protect you through fight-and-flight while the other uses an opposite strategy taking you into disconnection and collapse. Although both pathways are always available, over time your nervous system begins to depend more on one of these two strategies. I think of this as a home away from home—a place that offers refuge when home is not available. My home away from home is in disconnection and collapse. When life feels too challenging, I shut down and disappear.

Which survival strategy is your default? Fight-and-flight or disconnection and collapse?

Just like your home in regulation has a landscape with characteristics that define it, so does your home away from home. Close your eyes and imagine the landscape of the place you've identified as your home away from home. What do you see and hear as you look around? What are the features that define this place: colors, energy, shapes, objects, features of the natural world, structures, people, and animals?

Use this space to write about, or illustrate, your home away from home.

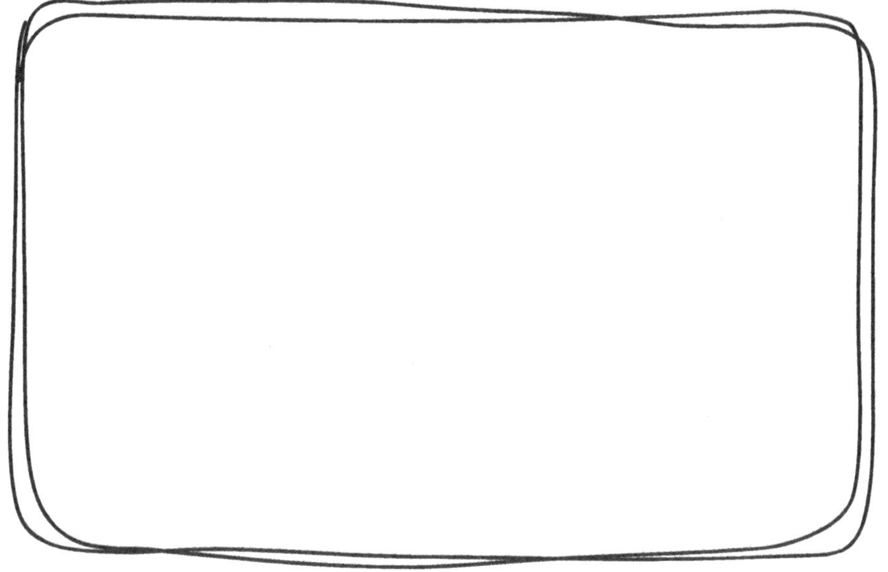

scan me!

To explore more about building your home away from home, listen to this Home Away from Home audio practice soundstrue.com/the-nervous-system-workbook-bonus.

flavors of states

States of regulation and dysregulation bring a variety of experiences and a wide variety of words to describe them. For example, some people talk about regulation as flow, calm, and focused, while others define it as excitement, purpose, and passion. The two pathways of dysregulation bring equally diverse flavors. Some of the common words that describe fight-and-flight are cranky, raging, worried, and panicked while shutdown is often labeled drained, lost, down, and hopeless.

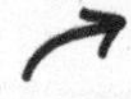

What words describe your experiences? Use these lists to find the words that describe the flavors of your states. Circle the words that fit and add any words you want that aren't listed.

Regulation	Fight-and-Flight	Shutdown
calm	angry	drained
peaceful	frustrated	lost
playful	raging	down
passionate	cranky	hopeless
zen	annoyed	despairing
relaxed	furious	collapsed
bliss	irritated	numb
flow	mad	foggy
focused	infuriated	discouraged
excited	aggravated	dejected
forthright	anxious	despondent
honest	worried	abandoned
quiet	nervous	alone
purposeful	scared	depressed
at ease	distressed	disconnected
	panicked	floating
	alarmed	invisible
	desperate	
	distracted	
	impatient	
________	________	________
________	________	________
________	________	________

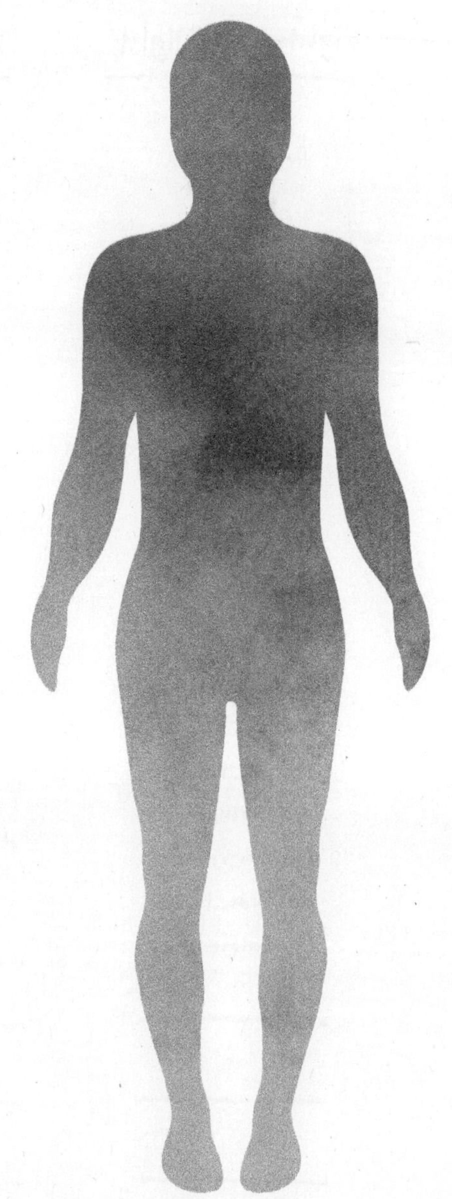

embodying my states

What happens in your body is an important source of information. How is the easy flow of energy in regulation felt differently from the intense energy of fight-and-flight or the draining of energy with collapse? How each appears in your body helps you tune into the signals coming from these states. These signals create the patterns that turn into familiar behaviors and stories and impact your daily life in significant ways. Recognizing how you embody regulation and dysregulation helps bring awareness to the patterns.

→ **Using this body drawing, write or draw where you feel each of the following energies:**

Where in your body do you feel the energy of *regulation*?

Where in your body do you feel the energy of *activation*?

Where in your body do you feel the energy of *shutdown*?

You might use colors to identify the places where each energy is felt.

→ **List the ways you feel each state.**

the gifts of survival states

A basic principle of the biology of the nervous system is that it is always working in service of your survival. From moment to moment, your nervous system assesses for danger and enacts a response. While at times your thoughts, feelings, or behaviors may seem irrational, the move into protection and the accompanying behaviors are simply your nervous system responding to the signals it's receiving with the goal of keeping you safe.

Reflect on a moment when the flood of fight-and-flight energy came to your rescue. For example, I was recently overwhelmed trying to navigate the healthcare system. It was a confusing nightmare, but rather than my usual response of giving up, I got angry and was able to persist until I got some answers. What are the ways your fight-and-flight energy worked to help you in the moment you've identified?

→ **Write a letter to this survival state to express your appreciation.**

Now reflect on a moment when you were saved by the pull into disconnection and shutdown. For example, I found myself feeling extremely anxious during an event I had to attend. While I was physically present, emotionally I went into "robot mode," going through the motions from behind an imagined plexiglass shield. It was my nervous system's way of helping me feel safe. How did disconnecting and shutting down help you in the moment you've identified?

Write a letter to this survival state to express your appreciation.

three things

We naturally create emotional connections with objects and assign meaning to them. We use their physical attributes to represent our feelings and tell a story. You can use this process to explore your nervous system. When you think about connection, activation, and disconnection, what objects come to mind? I love beach stones and am always looking for stones that evoke my experiences of connection, activation, and disconnection. I have a collection of heart-shaped stones that remind me of connection, stones with different colors for activation, and flat stones for disconnection. I have fun discovering objects that represent my states and I am always on the lookout for new ones.

Now it's your turn. Choose an object to represent each of your states—one for connection, one for activation, and one for disconnection. You might choose three objects from the same category like my beach stones, or you may find objects from different categories. Try out different objects and let your experience be your guide.

↗ **Use this space to write about your objects and why you chose them.**

Connection

Activation

Disconnection

becoming safely still

In the beginning, stillness may not bring a state of rest and renewal. Instead, for some, it can feel uncomfortable and cause anxiety. This is a normal and not uncommon experience. Over time, through the practice of coming into stillness, your capacity to rest in peace and quiet deepens and you'll begin to find comfort there. Each moment of stillness is a moment that nourishes your nervous system. When you learn to experience safety in stillness, you can be comfortable with silence, engage in self-reflection, attune with another person, meet them in wordless connection, and be present to the joy of intimate experiences. And once you find the words, people, and places that welcome you, you can intentionally invite moments of stillness into your daily life.

Lots of different words describe stillness—silence, quiet, serenity, tranquility.

→ **What word(s) describes your sense of being safely still?**

→ **Name the people with whom you can connect in moments of stillness. What is it about the relationship that makes it possible to share a moment of stillness?**

→ **Certain places in your daily life bring you the opportunity to enter a moment of quiet. Where are those places and what are the qualities that invite you into stillness?**

pathways to play

Play relies on the regulating and activating systems working together. I like to imagine these systems metaphorically holding hands, sharing their energy so we feel energized, safe, and ready to play. Whether you think of yourself as a playful person or see yourself as a serious problem-solver, playfulness is an essential ingredient of well-being and a quality that can be enhanced and become part of your daily lived experience. There are many ways to play. I love language, so every morning I get a word-of-the-day delivered to my inbox and then have fun trying to use it during the day. Recently my word was ensorcell (enchant, fascinate) and every time I used it, I had to define it! I also love social play and the playfulness of back-and-forth banter with friends, so I often bring that into my conversations. You can put play in motion with movement, play with objects including technology, engage in storytelling using your imagination to create a different sense of time and place, and play with others. Beyond adding a bit of joy to your day, moments of play help you to see new perspectives, expand your thinking, and manage challenges in new ways.

→ **Where, when, and with whom does your sense of playfulness emerge?**

→ **Where, when, and with whom does it disappear?**

→ **What are the ways you like to play?**

Use this information to create a plan in this box to bring more opportunities for play into your life.

my plan for play

in this moment

The nervous system is a dynamic system responding in every second with the energy you need to meet each moment and manage your day. Every day we all feel both subtle shifts in energy and the bigger shifts between connection and protection. When you take individual moments and bring them together, you can see the flow of your day. Looking at your day not as a single point in time but as a series of moments broadens your perspective so you don't get stuck seeing your day through the lens of just one experience.

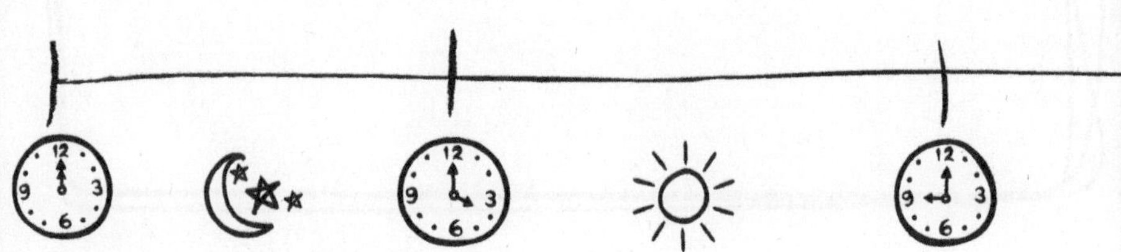

Use this timeline to describe your autonomic state at different times during the day. Was your energy regulated, activated, or disconnected?

Reflect on the autonomic path you traveled. What shifts did you experience today?

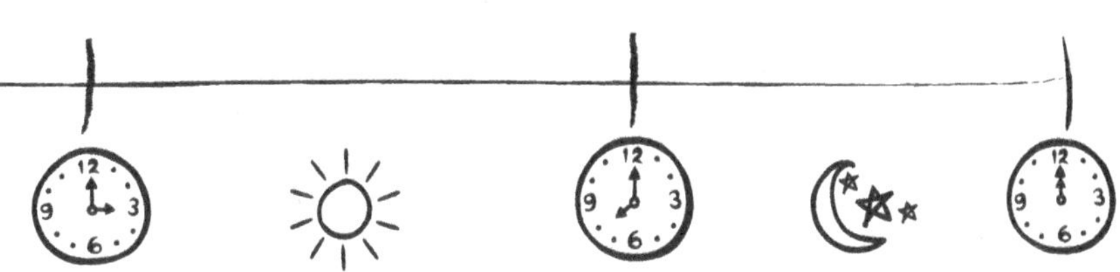

storytelling

Humans are storytellers by nature. We are driven to make meaning and it is through your nervous system that you first create, and then inhabit, your stories. The core beliefs you carry about yourself, others, and the world begin not in your brain but in your nervous system. Each of your autonomic states has its own set of messages and as you move from state to state, the storylines change. From collapse, the stories are about losing hope, not belonging, being unseen and alone. From the activation of fight-and-flight, the stories are ones of anger and anxiety, action and chaos. From regulation and connection, the stories are about possibility and choice, of feeling safe enough in the world to venture out and explore.

Read the following definitions of the three states—ventral connection, sympathetic activation, and dorsal collapse—and get to know how each state shapes your stories.

Regulated and Ready

When you are firmly grounded in your ventral pathway, you feel safe and connected, calm and social. From an anchor in regulation, you have the organization and resources needed to navigate your day with a bit of equanimity.

→ **Give your ventral state a name:**

____

→ **Now finish these sentences:**

I am ______________________________

______________________________.

The world is ______________________________

______________________________.

People are ______________________________

______________________________.

Anxious and Angry

When you are pulled into the flood of energy in sympathetic survival, you feel a flavor of danger, are ready to react, and are mobilized to respond. Here you travel the twin pathways of fight-and-flight, feeling the rise of anger and anxiety.

Give your sympathetic state a name:

____

Now finish these sentences:

I am ______________________________

______________________________.

The world is ______________________________

______________________________.

People are ______________________________

______________________________.

Down and Out

When you are pulled down into dorsal you move into shutdown. You feel drained, without enough energy to engage with the world. You collapse, disconnect, and disappear.

→ **Give your dorsal state a name:**

→ **Now finish these sentences:**

I am ______________________________.

The world is ______________________________.

People are ______________________________.

learning to listen

There are two different ways to listen: from the outside in and from the inside out. Each way offers a different pathway to awareness, allowing you to tune in to the elements that make up a moment in time and find your state. The following questions lead you to listen with curiosity and offer a way to practice coming into safe connection with your autonomic experience. This is an information-gathering practice, with a goal to find your state by going through the questions. There is no good or bad outcome, no good or bad state to be in. When you can listen to the elements that lead you to a state without judgment and with curiosity, you have taken an important step in befriending your nervous system.

Choose an experience to explore and follow the prompts for listening from the outside in.

Where am I? (Locate yourself in time and space.)

What's happening in my environment?

Who is around? What am I doing?

What state am I in? (regulated, fight-and-flight, or shutdown)

Choose another experience and follow the prompts below to listen from the inside out.

What am I sensing in my body?

Where is energy moving?

Where is energy not moving?

Do I feel filled?

Do I feel flooded?

Do I feel empty?

What state am I in? (regulated, fight-and-flight, or shutdown)

belonging

Belonging is not just a psychological state, it's a biological need. Safe, reliable times of connection with others are a necessary ingredient for a life of well-being. You feel a sense of belonging when you are with people you know, and who know you, in deep ways. Belonging invites reciprocity—you give and take, offer and receive. When you are missing a sense of belonging, your nervous system is easily moved into the survival strategies of activation and collapse. Moments of belonging bring you to the sense of regulation that comes with safe connection and help you stay anchored in that place of well-being.

→ **Circle the words that bring you a feeling of belonging.**

→ **Cross out any words that bring you a feeling of not belonging.**

→ **Use the blank spaces to add other words that make you feel welcome.**

kinship	attached	included
connected	joined	family
synchronous	combined	intertwined
blended	united	related
allied	linked	community
mutual	together	alike
______	______	______
______	______	______
______	______	______

i believe

The ability to connect and find regulation with others (co-regulation) and to regulate on your own (self-regulation) are essential factors in successfully navigating daily life. These are the two wings of well-being. What did you learn in your family about being able to count on others and about being on your own? You may still carry what you learned in childhood, or your experiences may have taught you something new. Your beliefs about regulating with others and by yourself impact when you reach for connection and when you muddle through life struggling on your own. Becoming aware of the beliefs behind your behaviors helps you assess what's working and what you might want to change. With awareness you can continue to use what feels supportive and change what is holding you back.

What do you believe about regulation? Write about it here:

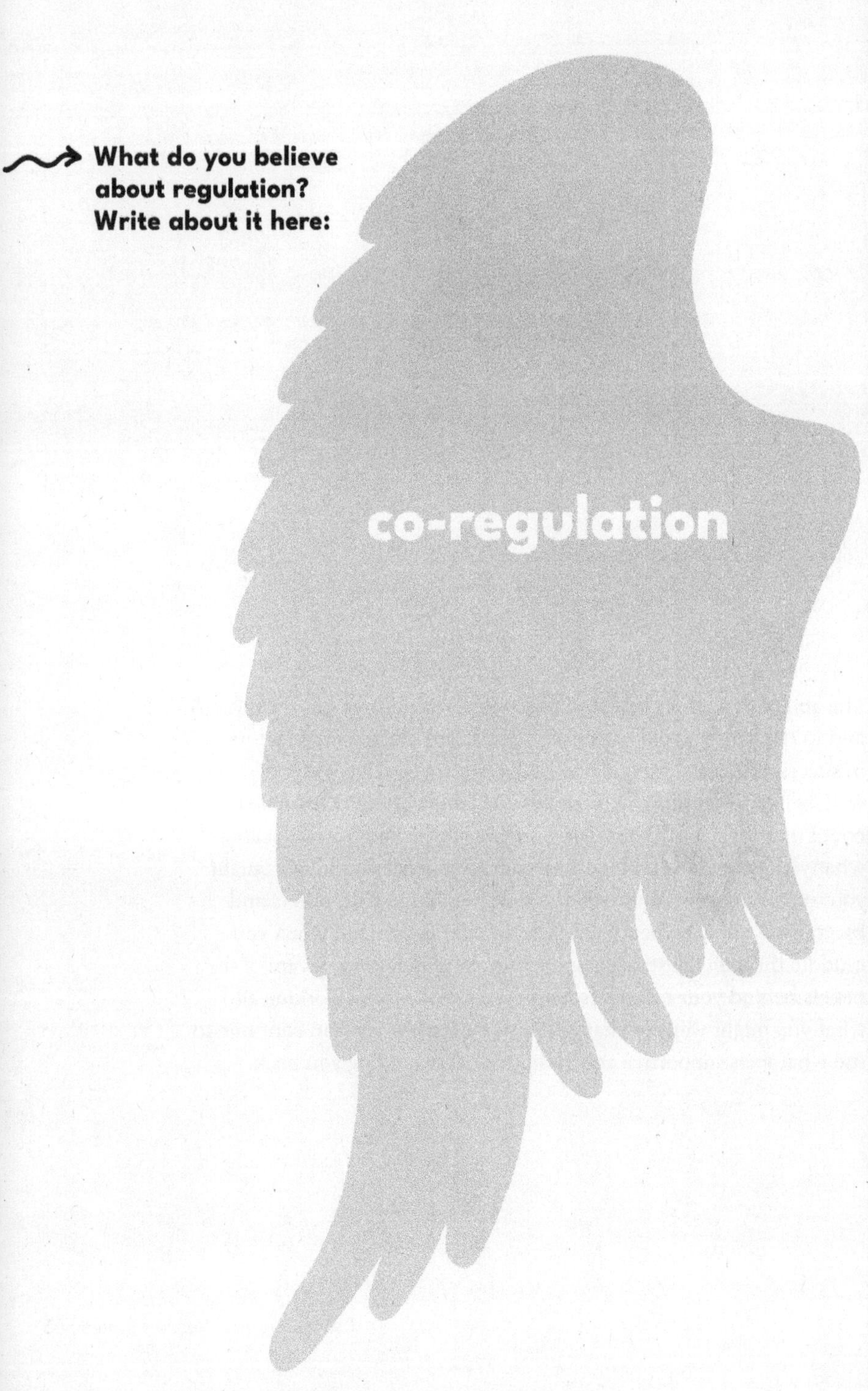

self-regulation

four pathways of connection

You're nourished by your essential connections to self, to others, to the world, and to Spirit. These connections are grounded in the nervous system. When you are anchored in regulation, the pathways welcome you and you can explore them with curiosity. Each of the four connections is important for well-being. The following practices will help you explore each pathway.

Connection to Self

You are not a single self but have many selves that have different thoughts about your daily experiences. It is common to talk this way in your daily conversations—there's a part of me that wants to visit my friend and a part that enjoys being alone. There's a part of me that wants to walk the beach and a part that wants to just sit and watch the waves. Your parts may have opposing ideas or similar ideas with different ways of enacting them.

Complete this sentence to see what inner connections you find:

There's a part of me that ______________________________

____

and a part of me that ______________________________

______________________________.

➔ Fill in more of these sentences and see what other connections you discover.

There's a part of me that ______________________________

____

and a part of me that ______________________________

______________________________.

There's a part of me that ______________________________

____

and a part of me that ______________________________

______________________________.

There's a part of me that ______________________________

____

and a part of me that ______________________________

______________________________.

Connection to Others

Who are the people in your life with whom you feel a connection? Think about your family, friends, coworkers, people in your community, and groups to which you belong.

What are the ways you connect with them? Do you see them in person or online? Do you make plans to meet or connect in spontaneous moments?

What are the things you do together that create and deepen connection?

Connection to the World

You connect to the world with the ways you inhabit space and move through the environment each day.

➔ **What are the characteristics of the places that feel welcoming and make you want to linger a bit longer?**

➔ **How can you describe the places you want to avoid?**

Connection to Spirit

Connection to Spirit comes in many forms and may be a well-traveled pathway or an emerging experience. There are a multitude of other words people use for Spirit including Goddess, Creator, Higher Power, Divine Being, to name a few, and many different ways to connect. For example, some people feel a spiritual connection when they are in nature, some when they enter a place of worship, and others in a moment of mindful contemplation. Connection can also happen through spiritual beings, spirit animals, energetic beings, and ancestral connections.

What word represents Spirit for you?

How do you connect with Spirit?

Close your eyes if you wish, open your heart if you can, and invite a connection to Spirit. Observe how it arrives for you in this moment. Reflect on your experience.

your pathways circle

When you bring the four connections together within a circle, in addition to seeing the individual pathways of self, other, the world, and Spirit, you see them in relation to each other and notice the balance or imbalance between them. You may discover that you rely on some pathways and rarely connect with others, or you may find that you travel the four pathways with similar frequency. Don't worry if your sections are unbalanced or some sections are less filled than others. Most people don't have a perfect balance and find one of the pathways is harder to access and less often used.

Note: This exercise uses colors, so you'll want crayons or markers.

First look at each of the four pathways of connection within the circle. Choose a color for each pathway and fill them in to represent how full or empty each one is.

Once your pathways are colored, notice which pathways you regularly rely on and which ones you use less often.

Looking at all four pathways together is a measure of your general sense of connection. Consider your circle as an integrated whole with four pathways that combine to nourish you.

What is your overall feeling of connection?

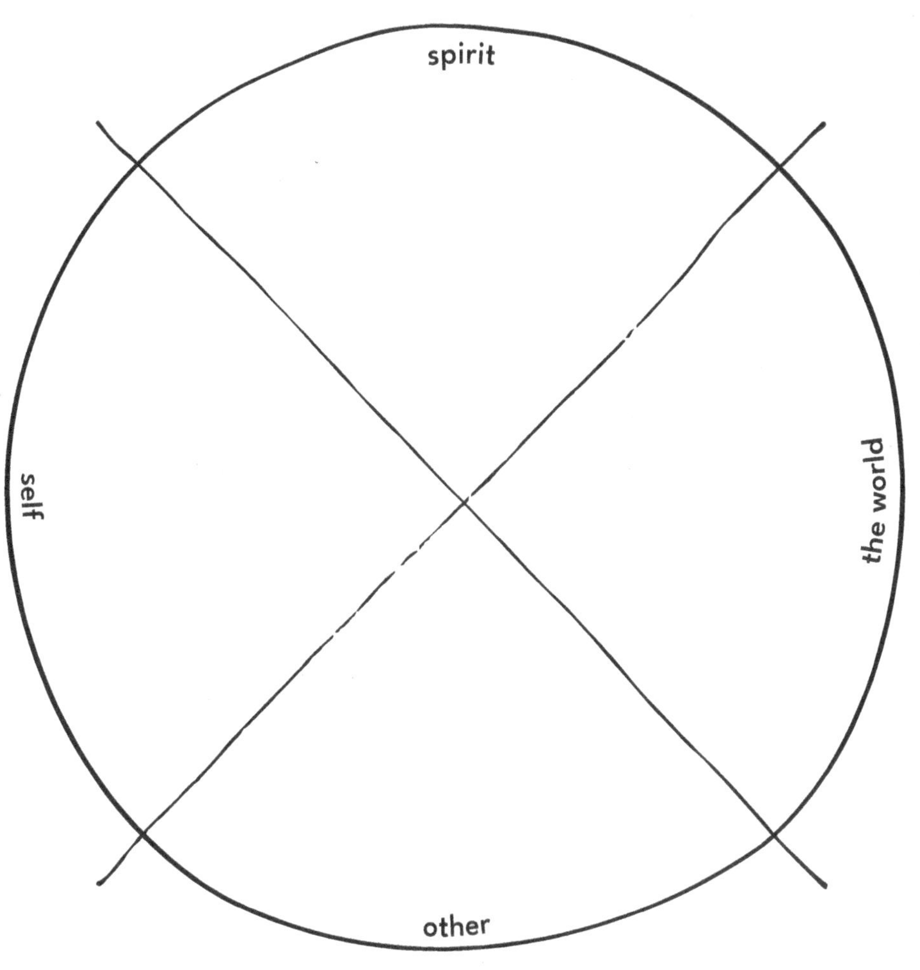
spirit
self
the world
other

my inner surveillance system

Your nervous system has a built-in surveillance system that watches for signs of safety and looks for warnings about dangers ahead. It broadcasts messages from below the surface of awareness. You might think of this embodied system as gut instinct or your autonomic intuition. When you bring awareness to this information system, and learn how it sends you messages, you can tune in and use the information to inform your decisions.

Let's do a body scan. You can close your eyes or do this with your eyes open, whichever feels most comfortable. Start with bringing attention to your feet and notice any feelings and sensations. Now gradually move upward to your head continuing to pay attention to feelings and sensations.

Look for the place where your own surveillance system lives.

Once you've found it, focus on that place in your body and invite an image to represent your surveillance system. Draw it here.

Now that you have your image, spend some time getting to know how it works. How does it track signs?

Now remember a time when your surveillance system alerted you. How did it send you signals?

inside, outside, between

Your nervous system works tirelessly to answer the question, "Am I safe?" It is always accessing information through three pathways:

- the inside pathway of embodied sensation
- the outside pathway that brings awareness of the world around you
- the between pathway that senses the dynamics in a relationship

Each of these pathways is continuously taking in information while looking for signs of welcome and warning.

Choose a moment you'd like to look at through the lens of these three pathways.

What signs were sent by each of your three streams—inside, outside, and between? Fill in these boxes with the signs of welcome and warning.

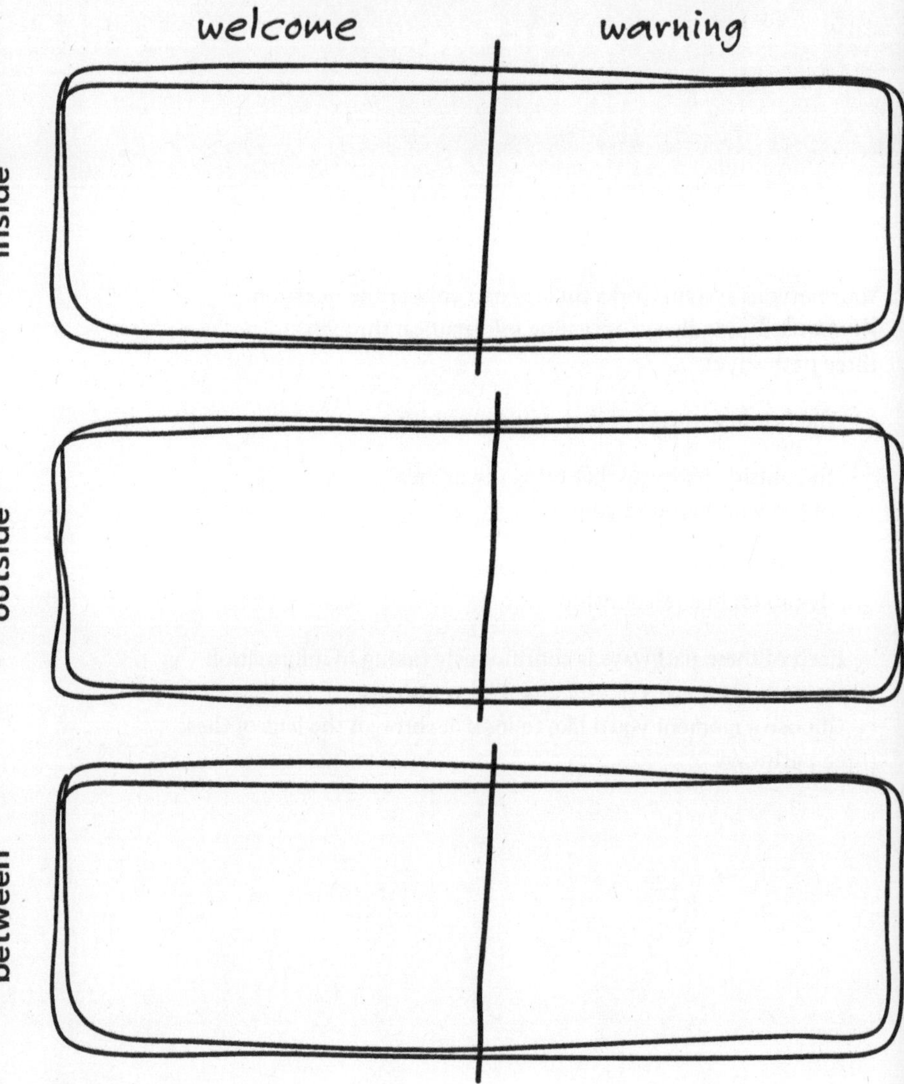

As you see your experience in this way, how did the signs of welcome and warning shape your experience?

an information pathway

Your behaviors, feelings, and stories are rooted in your nervous system. Knowing that your experiences begin in your biology helps you bring awareness to what otherwise remains hidden. From the place where you found your surveillance system, sometimes called gut feeling or intuition, you can take the next step and find the place where you locate perception. These two experiences, nervous system awareness and cognitive perception, combine and offer you a new and expanded pathway to follow in both directions. With this information you can track the sequence of your stories, actions, and feelings from cognition to their roots in your nervous system and back again. When you track your experiences in both directions and include these elements of your experience, your viewpoint expands and you can see what's happening from a different perspective.

Place one hand on the part of your body where you feel your surveillance system. Place your other hand on the part of your body where you find perception. Imagine the route between your two hands. Draw the pathway labeling the two ends. It might be a straight line between the two points or a more circuitous route. Now move along the pathway from surveillance to perception, adding one point for feeling and one for action.

Think of an experience when you clearly knew the story but aren't so sure how you got there. Using the pathway you drew, travel from perception backward to its roots in your nervous system. Begin at the perception end, then move to action, then feeling, before arriving at your surveillance system and identifying the sign of safety or danger that was at the very beginning of the experience. Jot down the story below.

Perception/story

Action

Feeling

Sign of Safety or Danger

Write this story, starting with your surveillance system's signs moving through feeling, to action, and finally perception.

This same sequence works in the opposite direction. This time choose a moment when your body sensations are easy to recall but you're not so sure about the story.

Sign of Safety or Danger

Feeling

Action

Perception/story

the world of sound

The world around you is a sonic environment with layers of sounds that affect your nervous system. Some sounds are welcoming and invite you to anchor in regulation while others challenge your ability to be present and prompt a move into protection. As you go through your day, you are traveling through an ever-changing soundscape.

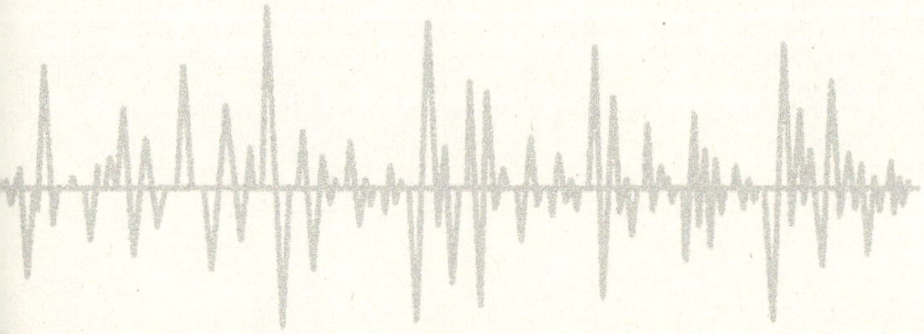

Tune into your soundscape.

→ **What are the sounds around you? Which ones invite you in and which ones bring a bit of discomfort?**

→ **As you move through your day, keep tuning in to the different soundscapes and noticing the sounds. Once you have collected a sample of sounds, notice which ones help you feel anchored in safety and connection and describe them here.**

→ **Imagine a place that brings these sounds together. Draw it or write about it and feel it come alive.**

my musical map

Music is all around you—a powerful and readily available regulator of the nervous system. Songs are a way to reach for regulation and touch survival states. Some songs deepen your experience of feeling safe and social while other songs let you embrace moments of anger, anxiety, and despair without feeling overwhelmed. When you listen to music you feel met, understood, and not alone. When you find the music that moves you, you access a practical and easy path to befriending.

- **Listen to all kinds of music using whatever device or subscription you use to access music and build a playlist with songs that evoke different flavors of connection and protection. Arrange them in an order that intersperses songs of safety with songs of survival and travel through these states with ease.**

- **It's also fun to create a playlist that only includes music that deepens your sense of safety and connection for times when you just want to rest in regulation or celebrate feeling anchored in safety.**

my playlists

my regulating resource menu

There is no right or wrong way—there is the way of your nervous system. This sentence is a reminder that everyone finds their own way to regulation. Every day you reach for resources to hold onto regulation and find the way back from moments of dysregulation. How you do that depends on your nervous system responses. When other people offer advice, or your friends share what they do, ask your nervous system if those suggestions fit for you. Try them out and see if they take you to regulation. If the answer is yes, add it to your list and if the answer is no, recognize that this is not a resource for you and move on.

A successful regulating resource menu needs to include a variety of resources. You might talk to a friend, take a walk, make a cup of tea, snuggle with your cat, attend a yoga class, or do a breathing practice. Some days you're drawn to a certain resource and other days you want something different. The list of resources is only limited by what brings you into regulation. Art, music, writing, nature, movement, breath, touch, people, pets, and technology are just some of the categories to explore. Certain places feel like a resource and even remembering past moments can rekindle regulation.

It's time to come up with your own regulating resources menu. Resources come in the categories of self-regulating and co-regulating so be sure to include things you do on your own and things you do with others. Remember, different resources demand different amounts of energy. Listening to music uses less energy than meeting a friend. Sitting somewhere that feels regulating is less demanding than going to the gym. Find a variety of resources for your menu so you have choices that will match the energy you have available when you need one.

Use this space to come up with your own resource menu.

part two

coming home to safety and connection

The wonderful thing about your autonomic nervous system is that it is always changing. Old patterns can be interrupted and new ones can be shaped. Your responses aren't set in stone. You can engage in practices that help you more easily find your way to safety and connection and spend more time feeling regulated and ready to engage with the world. You can shape your system in new ways and enjoy the sense of ease that comes from living with a nervous system that responds with flexibility to the ordinary—and sometimes extraordinary—challenges you meet each day.

The exercises in part 2 are designed to help you create greater capacity to anchor in regulation, expand your ability to feel safe, and navigate daily experiences in new ways. Some are here for you to use in the moment as you are looking for safety and others are a way to shape new pathways of connection. Each exercise, whether a resource to reach for in a moment of need or a way to proactively shape your system in the direction of connection, is an invitation to begin to become an active operator of your nervous system and the author of your personal stories.

anchoring in safety

Autonomic anchors are a reliable way to find a feeling of safety. They hold you when experiences threaten to overwhelm you and can help you find the way back from dysregulation to regulation and stay there. But they don't automatically appear. You first need to find them and then learn to call on them.

Anchors are found in connection with people you know, places you visit, and things you do.

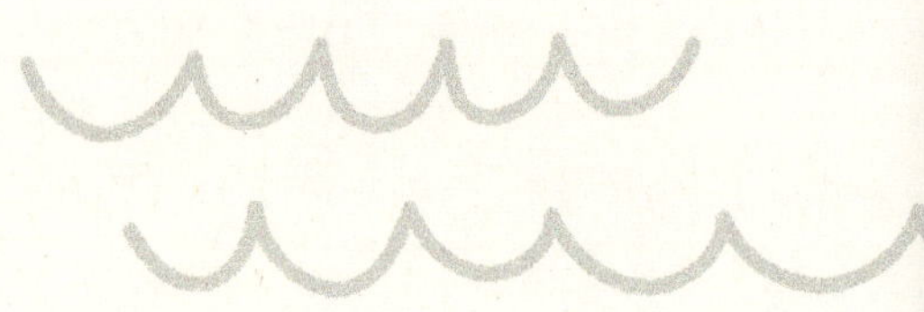

→ Who are the people in your life who bring you a sense of feeling safe and welcome?

You might also have a pet who fills this role. I have a childhood friend who is one of my anchors and a colleague who is another. And of course, my cat, Buddy, is always around ready for a snuggle.

→ Where are the places in your world that bring you a sense of belonging?

Think about the everyday places that you move through (home, neighborhood, nature, workplace, place of worship). The sea is my go-to anchoring place and even when I can't get there, the memory of being there brings me quickly to regulation.

↗ What are small things you do that feel nourishing and invite a sense of connection?

Look for things that are simple, quick, and easy to do in the flow of your day. I often take a moment to look out the window and see what's happening in nature or put my hand on my heart and connect with my breath.

Now that you've identified your anchors, make a habit of connecting with them. You can reach out and reconnect with your people or remember a moment of connection and feel anchored again in the energy of safety. The same is true for places you've identified—either revisiting or remembering will take you to regulation and safety.

When you engage in one of the actions you've identified as an anchor, you'll feel your nervous system respond. Remember, each time you reach for an anchor, you strengthen your capacity to return to regulation.

everyday safety

It's reassuring to remember that your everyday experiences regularly offer opportunities to anchor in safety. Often, the ordinary things you do—the things you're intuitively drawn to and that your nervous system naturally guides you toward—are regulating and the simple act of engaging with, and recognizing these, is nourishing. When you bring awareness to the ordinary things that have personal meaning for you, you can harness the power of these everyday experiences.

What do you wear that helps you feel wrapped in regulation? Do you have a favorite sweater, t-shirt, pair of shoes, hat, or piece of jewelry? Reach for those on the days you want to feel held in that energy. What scents evoke a sense of safety and connection? Find ways to bring those into your environment (essential oils, diffusers, candles, body cream). What objects remind you that you are safe? Put them in places you easily see. Find an object that is small enough to pick up and hold. Put it in your pocket and take it with you on a day that feels challenging.

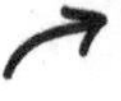

Take a moment and write down some of your ordinary objects that have the power to help you regulate.

awe inspiring

Feelings of awe fill us with wonder, stimulate our curiosity, and for just a moment take us out of our everyday lives into a moment of reverence and deep appreciation. In a moment of awe, we experience being in the presence of something vast that transforms our experience of the world. We feel like we are a single person connected to a community of people and connected to the planet.

Awe can be found in extraordinary moments. You encounter something amazing that stops you in your tracks, a moment so inspiring you are awestruck. Awe is also found in everyday experiences: a bird singing, a flower blooming in the garden, a piece of music playing. Moments of awe are abundant in our everyday world. Awe shapes the nervous system toward regulation. Finding small moments of awe contributes to an ongoing sense of well-being.

Remember a moment of awe.

Close your eyes and replay it in your mind and bring the richness of the moment back to life. Notice what happens in your body and the feelings that emerge. Listen to the story that accompanies the memory.

Notice the places where you regularly find awe—think of these as your awe environments.

Where are the places you can return to easily and find a moment of awe?

Small moments of awe add up and shape your system in the direction of connection and toward well-being.

→ **Write a one-sentence intention to help you remember to connect with the everyday moments of awe that are all around you.**

Mine is: I will watch for the moments of awe that appear in my day.

traveling regulated pathways

Back in the first prompt of part I, you learned about your system in balance. You discovered that when you're anchored in regulation your survival states give up their protective strategies of fight-and-flight and shutdown and instead work together to bring you a sense of safety and connection. We're going to use this knowledge now to sense the interconnection between your three states (ventral, sympathetic, dorsal) and imagine the pathway that allows you to travel between them with ease.

As you begin, remember there is an order to the ways your states connect—ventral leads to sympathetic which leads to dorsal.

Visualize a pathway that connects your three states and invites you to travel between regulation, the energy of aliveness, and the nourishment of rest and digest.

You might see a path to walk, stairs to climb, a series of bridges to cross, or a light stream to ride. Let your imagination loose and see what image appears. Notice any changes in your path as you move from state to state.

Describe or draw your pathway in this space with as much detail as possible:

Now that you've visualized and described or drawn your pathway, the next step is to travel along it. Close your eyes and imagine you are standing on your pathway. Then explore the journey that takes you from one end to the other. Change the image in any way you need to feel safe and able to move with ease.

What did you discover about traveling your regulated pathway?

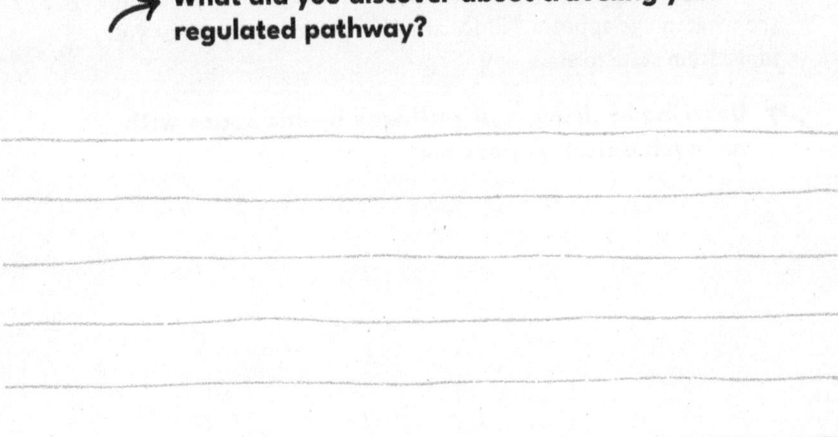

Daily life tip:

Return to travel your regulated pathway regularly. Each time you make the journey your body brings you a sense of well-being and your brain brings a story of safety and connection.

navigating survival pathways

Your survival pathways are more challenging to navigate than your regulated pathway. Instead of an interconnected pathway with states that work together, your survival states each have their own strategy and rather than an easy transition, the pathway from one to the next often feels disjointed. Intentionally connecting helps you begin to manage your move into protection and guide you back home to safety. You can learn to travel your survival pathways by becoming comfortable with how they work and confident in your ability to travel them, so they don't feel so scary and overwhelming. Each time you bring awareness to the experience of moving into survival and returning to regulation, you strengthen your ability to go from connection to protection and find your way back again.

While it may seem counterintuitive to intentionally leave regulation and enter survival energy, engaging in this exercise is a way to visualize the route from safety into survival states and add safeguards to make the experience more manageable.

Begin by imagining the pathway you take when you move out of regulation into the energy of fight-and-flight.

You might see a steep path, a rope ladder, stairs, or a beam of light. Take time to experiment with images until you find one that feels right to you. Then add elements to the image that help you manage the pace and keep you from simply free-falling into that survival state. You could add a place to rest, handholds, or a harness to hook into. Play with this until you create a way to slow the process, feel like you have some control, and aren't just automatically pulled into fight-and-flight.

Describe or draw your pathway with as much detail as possible:

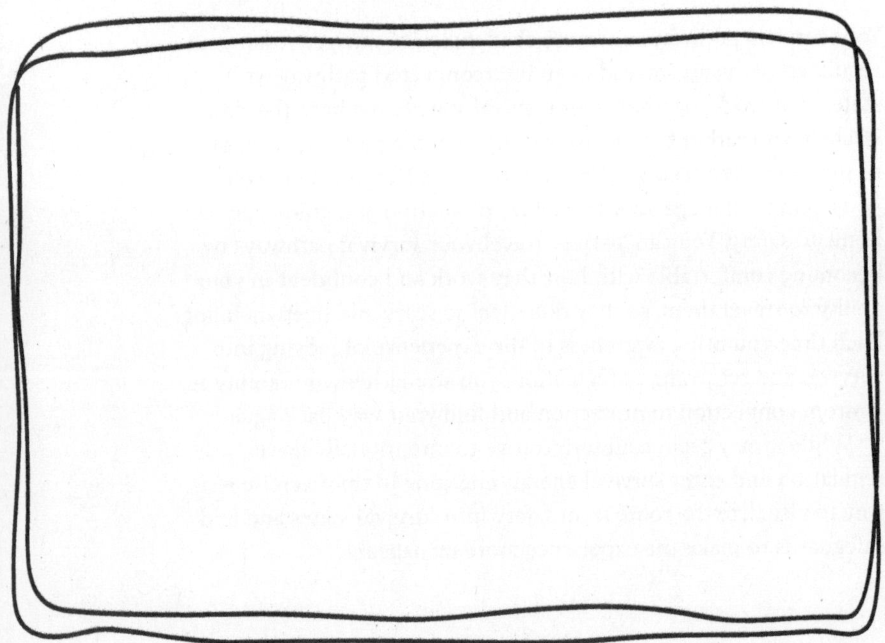

Now visualize the path that leads from fight-and-flight into shutdown.

It may be a continuation of the same path, or it may look very different. Add elements to the path that help you manage the descent and keep you from plummeting into collapse.

→ **Describe or draw your pathway with as much detail as possible:**

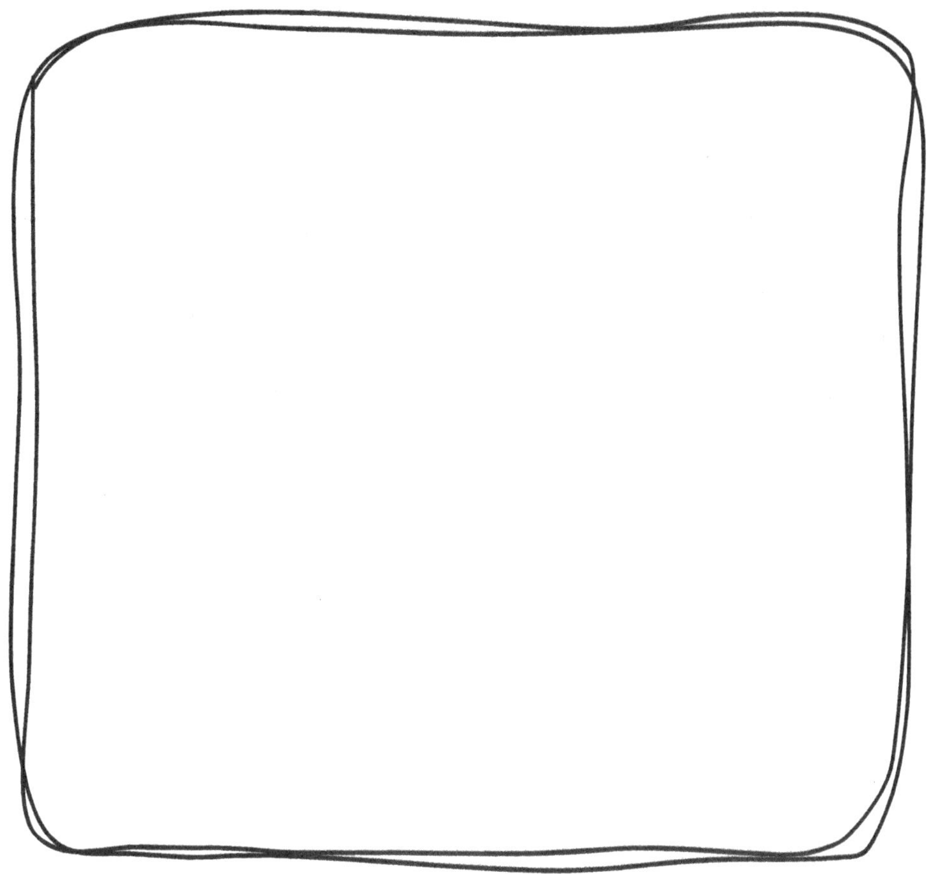

Finally, imagine the pathway that brings you back to safety and connection.

Visualize the route that takes you out of collapse, passes by fight-and-flight, and ends in regulation. Add whatever elements you need to be able to travel this pathway with some ease.

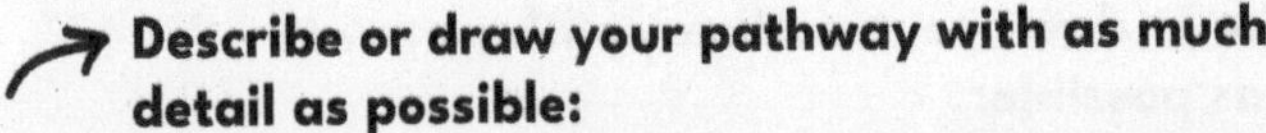

Describe or draw your pathway with as much detail as possible:

Revisit your pathways regularly and practice moving with intention out of connection without automatically falling into survival. Intentionally travel the pathway back to regulation. With practice, you can begin to respond less intensely, and recover more quickly when situations pull you out of regulation.

fillers and drainers

Daily life regularly brings moments that fill and moments that drain. Certain people, places, and actions feel nourishing while others feel depleting. The balance between fillers and drainers shapes your experience and contributes to your overall experience of a day. Making sure the drainers don't overwhelm the fillers is important for everyday well-being.

Let's get to know your personal fillers and drainers. How do you experience each?

Think back on a time when you felt drained. How did it show up in your body, your behavior, and your beliefs?

Now reflect on a filling experience. How did that show up in your body, your behavior, and your beliefs?

Reflect on a day from the recent past and list all the fillers and drainers you experienced in that day.

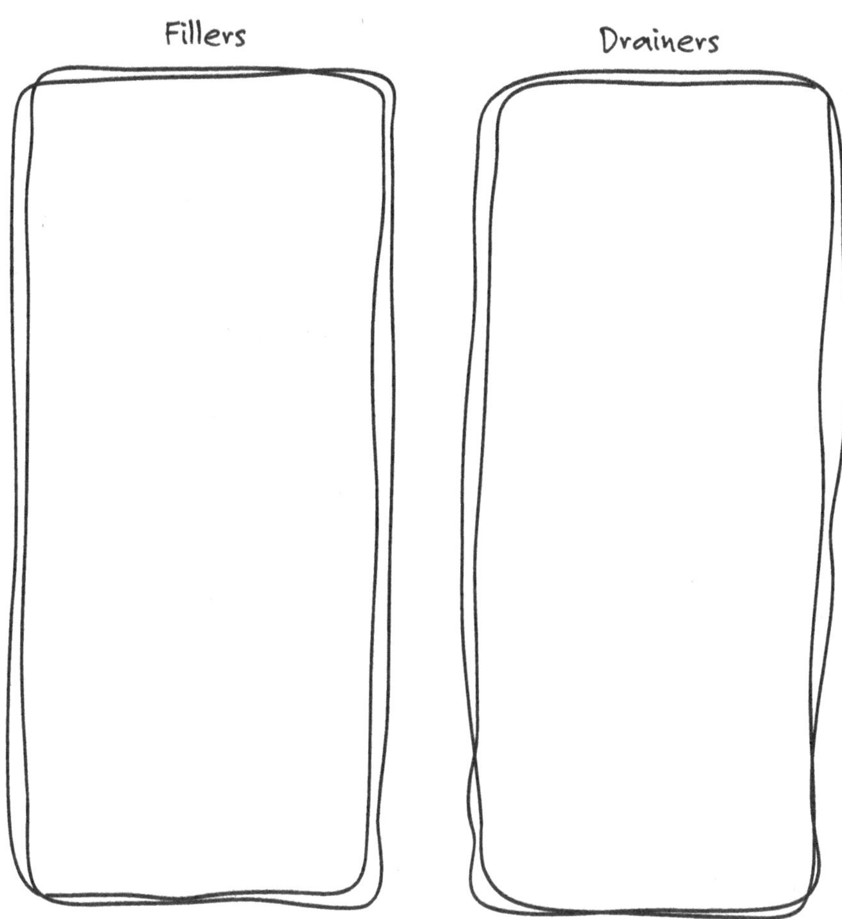

Now compare the lists. Would you call it a nourishing day or a depleting day?

just like me practice

This practice helps you move from a sense of being an individual different from everyone else—*me*—to a sense of being a part of the human family—*we*—by using statements that recognize the things that humans have in common. Everyone has a body, a mind, feelings, and thoughts, has suffered and experienced joy, and wants to be healthy and feel loved, just like you. When you engage with this practice you begin to see how other people's nervous systems are ordered, organized, and activated in ways just like yours. And when you see the similarities, you can move out of judgment and into compassion.

Here are some sentences I use:

Just like me this person can be warm and welcoming.

Just like me this person can disconnect and disappear.

Just like me this person can be pulled into anger easily.

Just like me this person can be regulated and invite connection.

Now write your own sentences.

Think about the ways you can feel safe, angry, anxious, and shut down; welcome others in; and shut people out.

Just like me this person can

Just like me this person can

Just like me this person can

Just like me this person can

Just like me this person can

Try this practice by starting with someone you're close to. Hold them in your awareness and say your sentences. Notice what feelings and stories emerge.

If you're ready to challenge yourself a bit, move to thinking about someone you are in a struggle with. Say your sentences and notice what feelings and stories emerge.

Create a habit of looking at people this way and over time you'll find it becomes easier to see others with compassion.

For more on building a sense of connection, listen to this Just Like Me audio practice soundstrue.com/the-nervous-system-workbook-bonus.

the art of savoring

Savoring is a way to make the most of a moment of safety and regulation. It is about seeing and celebrating the little things in everyday life. When we bring these moments into awareness and actively engage in attending to them, the benefits are both immediate, as we feel anchored in safety, and long term, with gains in physical and emotional well-being.

Do you remember the last time you ate something delicious, saw something beautiful, or felt a sensation of joy?

You might have thought, "How do I hold onto this feeling?" The art of savoring is a way to do just that. Savoring helps you hold a moment of goodness in conscious attention for up to thirty seconds to amplify its effect. While savoring is meant to be a way to deepen positive moments, it's easy for negative thoughts to intrude and interrupt the deepening practice. Common negative thoughts include, "I don't deserve to feel good. If I feel good something bad will happen. It's not fair that I can feel this way when other people are suffering." What are the negative thoughts you most often hear? If a thought interrupts your savoring, simply stop the practice and try again later. Over time, you'll get better at the practice and the dampening thoughts will appear less often. Once you begin to practice, you'll regularly discover moments during the day that you want to stop and savor.

Follow this Triple A method to stop and savor a moment at any time, in any place.

Attend: Notice a moment of safety, connection, or regulation. You can stop in real time as a moment happens or look back on your day and choose a moment.

Appreciate: Hold the moment in your awareness and appreciate its presence.

Amplify: Stay with the moment for 20–30 seconds. Soak in the sights, sounds, sensations, and story surrounding it.

It's great to have a place to keep track of your savoring moments. You could keep track in a "joy journal," keep a running list in a notebook, or add a note to each day on your calendar. What works for you?

It's also fun to have someone to share your savoring moments with. When you share your moments with another person, they come alive and you are filled with the energy of safety and connection.

Who could you invite to be a savoring partner with you?

Let's try it now. Use the space below to create a joy entry and then share it with someone.

SIFTing

SIFT is an acronym for body sensation, image, feeling, thought. The SIFTing practice uses these four elements as a way to remember and relive a moment of regulation. Similar to the idea of savoring, SIFTing helps us go even deeper with holding onto moments of joy and connection. As you create your SIFT, you return to the state of safety and connection that was present in the moment and strengthen your capacity for regulation.

→ Decide on a moment to SIFT.

Just as you did with savoring, choose a time when you felt regulated. You might have been feeling happy, at ease, peaceful, joyful, playful, or any other emotion that comes when you feel safe.

Write a short statement for each of these prompts.

What was happening in your body?

Sensation ______________________________

What is the image?

Image ______________________________

What are your feelings as you are back in the memory?

Feeling ______________________________

What is the thought that ties it all together?

Thought ______________________________

Give your SIFT a title.

You title should be a couple of words that represent the moment. Some of my favorites are Sand Dollar Beach, Gentle Rain, and Buddy and Me.

Title ______________________________

Read the title and four elements and settle into the memory of the moment. Let each element fill you and feel yourself back in the moment.

You can use this format to create a collection of SIFTs and reach for one anytime you want to anchor again in safety. These moments are already wired into your body-mind memory and are ready for you to return to whenever you want.

between stretch and stress

Have you ever thought you needed to take a break but didn't heed that warning and made a mess of what you were doing? Have you ever told yourself it was okay to not finish a job in one day but pushed yourself anyway to get the job done and ended up feeling sick the next day? When you feel as if you need to power through an experience or suffer to see results, you are stressing your nervous system and overlooking the signs that you are dysregulated. You are no longer acting out of a desire to change but from a fear of failing and you stay stuck in old patterns. Moving in a new direction requires you to stretch by trying something a bit different. The goal is to challenge yourself in the moment in a way that keeps you feeling regulated while reaching for something new—a new behavior, a new response, a new story.

The stretch-to-stress chart is a good way to recognize when you are in a positive change process and when you have pushed beyond your limits and instead of making a change, are now reinforcing old habits.

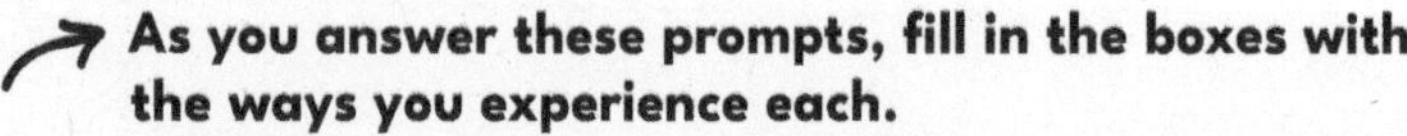

As you answer these prompts, fill in the boxes with the ways you experience each.

- What is it like in the stretch spot where you're shaping your system in some small new way? How does your autonomic nervous system let you know it is supporting you in this process, on board with making a change?

- Appreciate and notice what it feels like to stop for a moment and take in the change. What are the signs you are settling into a new pattern?

- Explore the stress spot and get to know the flavors of this experience. How do you recognize you've pushed too hard and you're no longer shaping a new pattern?

- Move to the survive spot. How do you recognize you are now reinforcing old habits and are stuck in a familiar pattern of protection?

Knowing the signs of stretch, appreciate, stress, and survive helps you make choices that support making changes. Return to this exercise when you are pushing too hard or when you need help supporting the kind of challenge that leads to change.

For more on Stretch and Stress, listen to this Both/And Shaping audio practice soundstrue.com/the-nervous-system-workbook-bonus.

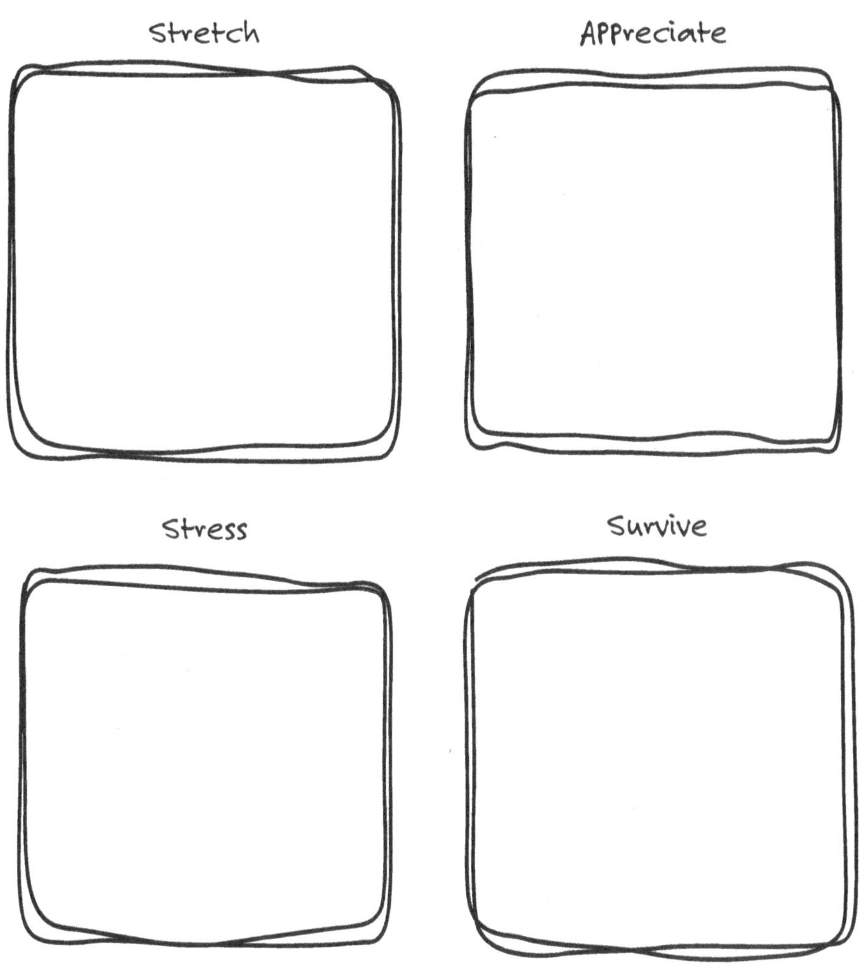
Stretch
Appreciate
Stress
Survive

disrupt and deepen

Anchoring in safety begins with awareness. With an attitude of friendship and an intention to befriend, you can engage with your nervous system and discover the patterns that are creating distress and deepen the ones that are nourishing.

Reflect on your daily routine. What patterns are no longer serving you? Maybe you stay up too late, drink more coffee than you should, spend too much time on social media, have trouble setting limits, or say yes when you really want to say no.

→ **Think about the past week and see what patterns are getting in your way.**

What patterns do you want to deepen? Do you have a good sleep routine, enjoy connections with friends, regularly find moments to play, or have a mindfulness practice?

→ **Think about the past week and see what patterns are supporting your well-being.**

Look at your list of positive patterns and take a moment to celebrate! Look at the list of patterns you want to change and don't worry. Recognizing patterns that aren't serving you is the first step to creating new patterns of well-being.

discernment

Have you ever looked back on an interaction and thought, "Wow, I really overreacted" or felt bad about the way you responded to an event and aren't even sure why you acted that way? A response that feels out of proportion to the event—a reaction that seems too big or too subdued—is often a cue from your past being brought to life in the present. You might fly into a rage when you spill your coffee, panic when you hear a car horn, or shut down when someone around you speaks in a loud voice. Other responses feel like they're anchored in the present and attuned to the moment. You get frustrated when you burn dinner, worry about being late when you're stuck in traffic, and go off by yourself when the people around you start to argue. It's helpful to know when your responses come from the past and when they are grounded in the present.

Look back on some recent experiences and choose a moment you're curious to explore to see if your response was in proportion to what was needed in the moment.

Notice we use the word *needed* and not *appropriate* since the nervous system doesn't assign meaning or motivation but simply enacts a response based on its assessment of safety. Write about that experience here.

Now ask yourself, "In that moment, in that place, with that person/people (if you were around others), was my level of response needed?" If the answer is yes, you were likely anchored in the present moment and your response was helpful in guiding your decisions.

Take a moment to acknowledge how your nervous system supported you.

If the answer is no, see if you can find a cue from your past that took you out of the present moment and into an old response. Maybe there was something in the environment that reminded you of a past danger or a way another person looked, spoke, or moved that was a reminder of someone who felt unsafe in some way.

Write down any of the cues of danger you find that are similar between the past and present.

Create a habit of using this discernment practice to assess an experience. This can be challenging when you're reacting to a moment and easier to build a practice of looking back on a moment and reflecting on your response. Over time you'll get good at recognizing the things that reach out to you from the past and aren't needed in the present, and find it easier to move in a new direction.

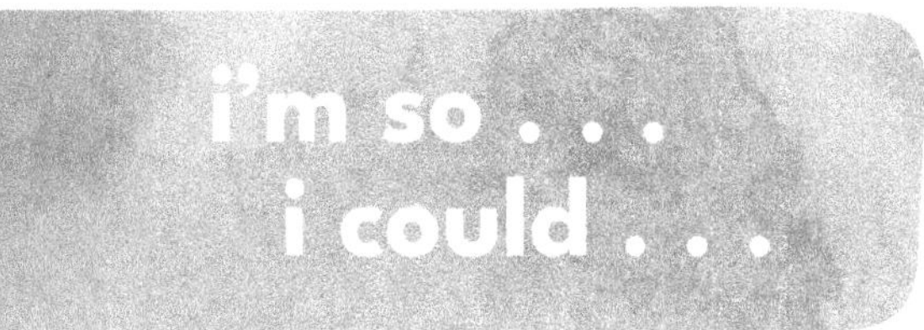

We often have a thought that follows the sentence structure,

"I'm so ______ [feeling], I could ______ [action]."

For example, "I'm so tired, I could give up." "I'm so angry, I could scream." "I'm so anxious I could run out of the room." "I'm so happy, I could smile at the world." With each of these sentences, your nervous system is sending you a message. The first emerges from a place of collapse, the second comes from the energy of fight, the third from the energy of flight, and the last from a place of regulation and connection. When you recognize the survival patterns, you can begin to gently shape them toward safety. When you notice the moments of regulation, you can anchor more firmly in connection.

Now it's your turn. Write four sentences of your own.

From disconnection and collapse:

I'm so ______________, I could ______________.

From anger:

I'm so ______________, I could ______________.

From anxiety:

I'm so ______________, I could ______________.

From safety and connection:

I'm so ______________, I could ______________.

Now, keeping the beginning of each sentence the same (I'm so), write a new ending (I could) for each.

What is a different response you could try out that would help shift you out of disconnection and collapse, soften the intensity of your anxiety or anger, and deepen your sense of safety and connection? For instance, "I'm so tired, I could give up" can be changed to "I'm so tired, I could rest for a bit." "I'm so angry, I could scream" can become "I'm so angry, I could walk away and cool off." "I'm so anxious, I could run out of the room" can become "I'm so anxious, I could look around the room for a friendly face." And "I'm so happy, I could smile at the world" might change to "I'm so happy, I could reach out and spend time with friends."

From disconnection and collapse:

I'm so ______________, I could ______________.

From anger:

I'm so ______________, I could ______________.

From anxiety:

I'm so ______________, I could ______________.

From safety and connection:

I'm so ______________, I could ______________.

This is a quick and easy way to look at a pattern and begin to shape it in a new way. As you hear yourself saying

"I'm so ______________, I could ______________"

take that moment to turn toward the first part of the sentence, bring a bit of regulation, and look for a different ending.

if/then

If/then statements help you plan when, where, and how you can respond to a situation. They bring awareness to experiences by creating a link between cues and responses making it easier for you to recognize situations that are dysregulating and take action. If/then statements work with people, places, and events that challenge your ability to stay regulated.

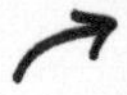

Think about a situation where you find it hard to stay regulated.

How would you like to respond differently? Use the framework "If this happens, then I will" to set a goal.

For example:

People **If** I'm going to be around family members who tend to stress me out, **then** I will make sure I have a touchstone in my pocket where I can reach it easily.

Place **If** I'm in a room that feels too crowded **then** I will make sure to stand near the door.

Event **If** my work to-do list feels overwhelming, **then** I will divide it into smaller parts and make sure to take a quick break every hour.

Now it's your turn.

People:

If ______________________ happens then I will:

____

Place:

If ______________________ happens then I will:

____

Event:

If ______________________ happens then I will:

____

If/then statements also work in situations where you feel safe and connected and want to deepen that experience. For instance:

People **If** I am with an old friend **then** I will tell them how much our friendship means to me.

Place **If** I am out in nature **then** I will stop for a moment to notice the beauty.

Event **If** I had a productive workday **then** I will celebrate that by adding a star to my calendar.

Now think about a situation you'd like to strengthen and use the if/then framework to set a goal.

People:

If ______________________ happens then I will:

____

Place:

If ______________________ happens then I will:

____

Event:

If ______________________ happens then I will:

____

tune in, take in, tend to

One of the ways to nourish your nervous system is with the three steps of tuning in, taking in, and tending to. The goal of this practice is twofold: notice when you are moving into survival and see what's needed to find your way to regulation, and recognize when you're anchored in safety and deepen the experience. The first two steps—tuning in and taking in—connect you to what is happening in your autonomic nervous system and the third step—tending to—uses that information to guide your actions.

Tune in What state you are in right now? Are you feeling safe and regulated? Anxious or angry? Disconnected or shut down?

Take in Look for cues of safety and danger. What do you sense in your body? What's happening in your environment? How do you feel about the people around you?

Tend to If you are dysregulated, what could you do to move toward safety and regulation? If you are feeling safe and connected, what could you do to stay there a bit longer? What would your nervous system tell you it needs to feel nourished in this moment?

return, reflect

Well-being is not defined by a nervous system that is always in regulation. A nervous system that brings qualities of well-being still dysregulates but rather than remaining stuck in a survival response, finds the way back to regulation. What small shifts have you already experienced today? Were there big shifts that took you between safety and survival? Take a moment to reflect on the autonomic journey that has brought you to this moment in time. As you nourish your nervous system and create more capacity for safety and connection, trust that you can react, return to regulation, and reflect on the experience. And trust that this is a sign of a healthy nervous system.

Try these three steps with a moment from your day.

React Recall a moment that had some intensity for you. Consider how you reacted. Where did your nervous system take you?

Return to regulation Remember the feeling of coming back to regulation and anchor there.

Reflect Think about the experience. What is there to learn from the way your nervous system responded?

getting unstuck

Feeling stuck in a challenging pattern that you can't seem to move out of is a common experience. Moving, either with actual physical movement or moving in your imagination, is a good way to get to know your sense of being stuck and offers a pathway to getting unstuck. Using repetitive movements such as clenching and unclenching your hand or walking in a circle can help you feel the physical sense of being stuck and tune in to the feelings and stories that accompany that experience. When you break the pattern by making a small change to your movements, your feelings and stories will change too.

→ **Decide on a pattern you feel stuck in and want to change.**

Create a movement pattern that represents your sense of being stuck.

This could be as simple as alternating pushing and pulling with your arms, turning your head from side to side, or pacing back and forth. Play with a few movements and see what fits your feeling of being stuck. A particularly memorable movement for me was stepping forward and back over and over, stuck in one place, never actually getting anywhere.

Enter into the movement pattern (either in your imagination or with actual movement) and repeat it several times.

What feelings emerge? What is the story you hear?

Experiment with changing the movement in some way. Interrupt the repetitive pattern.

In my example above, the way I interrupted the pattern was to stop stepping forward and back and step to the side instead.

What happens to your feelings, and your story, as you move in a new way?

Go back and forth between the two movements and feel how you can move between being stuck and unstuck.

breathe into safety

Regulation and safety happen when the heart and the breath are in harmony. Breath is regulated by your nervous system. It's an automatic process, but one you can also intentionally manipulate. As you bring attention and intention to your breath, you begin to shape your system toward safety.

Follow your breath Find the places where you feel breath moving in your body. Some of the usual places you may find your breath are the abdomen, chest, heart, throat, just under the breastbone, in the side ribs, in your lower back. Choose two places and put one hand on each. As you inhale and exhale, feel your breath moving between your hands. In your mind, follow the pathway of your inhalation and exhalation for a few breath cycles.

Add words Add intention to your breath by adding words to accompany each inhalation and exhalation. What do you invite in as you inhale and release as you exhale? I often choose to breathe in presence and breathe out worry, or breathe in joy and breathe out pain. What words work for you? Do you want to keep using these words or does each inhale and exhale bring new ones?

Invite movement Invite a movement to emerge as you inhale. Next, explore a movement that accompanies your exhalation. For example, I open my arms as I breathe in and pull them together in front of my heart as I breath out. Now join your two movements with your breath cycle and feel your body and breath moving together.

↗ **Reflect on your experience with breath and write down what you want to remember and return to.**

listen to the stories of your states

Through the lens of the nervous system, subtle shifts in your autonomic states translate into new stories about who you are and how you navigate the world. Humans are storytellers, meaning-making beings, and it is through your autonomic nervous system that you first create, and then inhabit, your stories. The information that begins in your biology travels autonomic pathways to the brain, where the brain creates a story to make sense of what's happening in the body.

From a state of collapse the stories have a flavor of losing hope, not belonging, feeling lost and alone. From a state of fight-and-flight, the stories are rooted in anxiety and anger, action and chaos. And from a state of regulation, the stories are ones of connection, possibility, and feeling safe enough to engage with the world. As your state changes, so do your stories.

Choose a small, ordinary experience you're curious about and feels just a bit challenging.

Connect with your state of collapse and shutdown. Listen to your experience from that perspective. What is it saying?

Connect with your state of fight-and-flight. Listen to your experience from that perspective. What is it saying?

Connect with your state of safety and regulation. Listen to your experience from that perspective. What is it saying?

intention setting

Setting an intention is a common practice in the process of making a change. Whether it is something small like wanting to take a daily walk or something bigger like looking for a new job, setting an intention is a way to stay connected to your goal.

When you write an autonomically informed intention, you invite your brain-based intelligence and your nervous system–based wisdom to work together. When your brain and body are not on the same page, your intention can create cues of danger and shut down your ability to follow through. You may have a desire to do something new or do something in a new way but an unrealistic expectation about how you are going to do that. For instance, I want to begin to walk regularly. My brain tells me to walk every day at 8:00 a.m. while my nervous system says that varying the times and walking several times a week might be more realistic. It's necessary to set an intention that brings the right degree of challenge—too bland and you'll get bored and too big and you'll be overwhelmed. The right-sized intention will catch, and keep, your interest.

What do you want to set an intention around? Is there a change you want to make or a pattern you want to deepen? Maybe you want to spend less time on social media, eat less sugar, or stick with your mindfulness practice.

Write your intention here.

Now read it out loud to yourself. Does it feel doable?

Change the words in any way you need to create an intention that you feel confident you can follow through with—an agreement that keeps you on the stretch side of the chart you created on page 123. Write your revised intention here.

Now that you have an intention that works for you, decide on how you are going to use it. I have a notebook for intentions and I read one each morning. Other people use their phones to record their intention and listen to it each day. Some people like to revisit their intention in the morning and others in the evening. What works for you?

As you begin to use your intention, take time to regularly reflect on the way your intention is becoming reality—the ways you are inviting the change you want into your daily life.

re-storying

As you gently shape your system in new ways and deepen into the nourishing patterns of connection, you naturally move into a time of re-storying—of attending to the autonomic shifts that are happening and weaving them into a new narrative. When you tune in to what is present, make a small change, and then tune in again, you can see how your story is being shaped in a new way. Imagery and words are two ways to hear your stories and write new ones.

→ **Let's start with imagery. Using imagery is a way to bring awareness to changes and hear the messages that accompany new patterns.**

Remember a moment of protection or connection and find an image to represent it. Write or draw the story below.

Include color, sounds, smells, a sense of energy, living things, and any other elements that are needed to complete the image and bring the moment alive. When you feel the image is fully formed, listen to the story it has to tell you. Write the story below.

→ Now, make a small change to the image.

Change one detail, one thing that might increase your feeling of safety and regulation. I often begin by changing colors and adding an object from nature. What do you want to add? What's the story now?

Change one more detail and listen in again.

Continue to play with changing one small detail and listening to the new story. Stop when you feel you've stretched far enough and going further would take you into feeling stressed. Reflect on the ways your story has changed.

Now let's try working with words. In the simple practice of changing just a word or two, you can listen to the beginnings of a new story. For this practice you'll work with statements about both protection and connection.

→ **First write a sentence that describes a state of protection.**

For example, "Relationships are dangerous and I'm better off on my own."

→ **Now change a word or two and write a new sentence that shifts the meaning toward the possibility of connection.**

For instance, "Relationships are dangerous and I'm better off on my own" can be changed to "Some relationships are dangerous and sometimes I'm better off on my own." Use words that add a different feeling to a sentence like *some, sometimes,* or *often,* and begin to reshape a story.

Now write a sentence inspired by a belief about safety in connection.

Change a word(s) and write a new sentence that deepens the experience.

Look for words that strengthen the feeling you've identified. For example, "I'm anchored in safety and connection" can be changed to "I'm firmly anchored in safety and connection."

With just a few small changes to images and adding a couple of words, you have the power to write a new story—one that brings you to safety and connection.

creating your resilience continuum

Moving out of regulation is a normal and expected experience. None of us are anchored in regulation all the time and the key to well-being is being able to return to regulation following moments of dysregulation. This ability to return is the essence of resilience. Resilience is not a stable quality. It ebbs and flows depending on your physical health, the number of demands you're trying to meet, and the amount of social support and connection you have. Tracking resilience is an ongoing activity. How resilient you feel guides how you respond to the challenges in your daily life, and the number and kinds of challenges and resources in your daily life impact your capacity for resilience. A resilience continuum is a good way to track your changing levels of resilience.

Draw a line in whatever shape you want to represent your resilience continuum. Label the two ends.

One end is where you feel an absence of resilience and the other end is where you feel an abundance of resilience. I call my two points "no energy and no interest" and "resilient and ready."

Identify three or four points between the two ends, name those places, and add them to your line.

I move from no energy and no interest to noticing, considering, curious, and then reach resilient and ready.

Now find your place on your continuum. Where are you in this moment?

How resilient are you feeling? Knowing where you are gives you information about what to do next. If you are on the resilient side of your continuum, you have access to all the qualities of a regulated system. You may want to move a bit further along the continuum or you may be content to stay right where you are. In either case, take some time to enjoy the feeling of regulation and resilience. When you find yourself on the non-resilient end of your continuum, reach for one of the resources you've created in earlier exercises. Remember you are building resilience each time you move back toward regulation.

creating your self-care circle

Do you regularly make time to take care of yourself? Or do you feel selfish when you focus on your own needs and have to justify doing things that bring you joy? Self-care means paying attention to your physical and emotional needs and taking steps to meet those needs. Practicing self-care is an ongoing, unfolding work in progress. When it comes to the nervous system it's important to listen, tend to what is nourishing, and follow what you are curious about. This is not a static activity. When self-care is guided by the nervous system, the question to ask is, "What am I doing to nourish my nervous system?" Attending to this question is the foundation for creating sustainable, autonomically sensitive self-care practices. Self-care emerges from the variety of options that bring your system of regulation alive. Your self-care circle reflects your changing needs and changing practices.

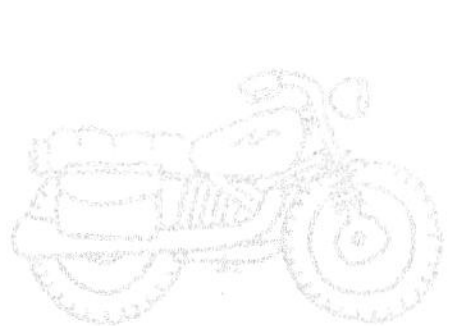

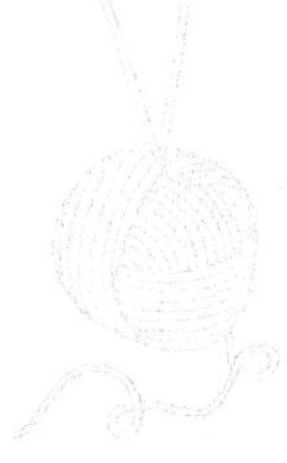

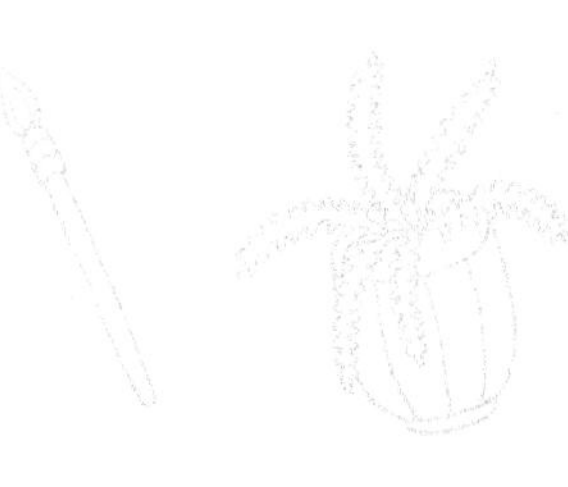

The self-care circle uses four categories—relational, spiritual, physical, mental—to explore things you are doing regularly in service of self-care and consider things you might like to try. What you are doing now goes inside the circle. What you want to try goes outside the circle.

Fill in each quadrant with activities you typically engage in that feel regulating and connecting.

If something feels like an activity you should do rather than want to do, or is a habit that doesn't bring you joy, don't add it to your circle.

Next, explore the space outside the circle.

What activities feel interesting that you'd like to try? Add these to the space outside the circle.

As you engage in the activities you've identified inside your circle and play with the ones on the outside, your self-care circle will change. Update it regularly. Remember: what you are drawn to and get joy from isn't set in stone and your changing self-care circle will reflect that.

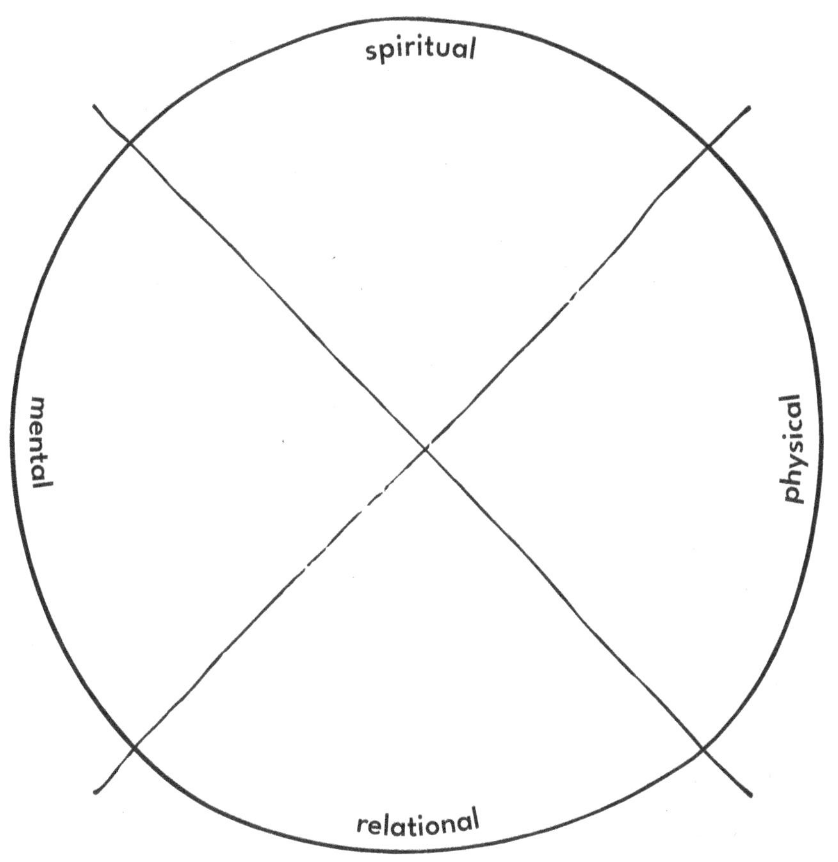
spiritual
mental
physical
relational

guiding questions

In each moment your nervous system is assessing for risk and safety. Your system has an inherent longing for safety and knows how to find the way there. From an anchor in safety, you experience the physical and psychological results that come from having a regulated nervous system. Strengthen your capacity to return to regulation and increase the time you spend there.

Make a practice of asking yourself these simple questions:

→ **What state am I in right now?**

If you are not in a place of regulation, ask yourself:

→ **What do I need to move toward safety?**

If you are in a place of regulation, ask yourself:

→ **What will help me stay here?**

passion and purpose

When feeling safe and connected becomes familiar and, on most days, regulation is easy to reach for, thinking about what you are passionate about and your purpose in life is a natural next step.

Passion becomes easier when you are anchored in safety and connection. From fight, flight, or shutdown, you are unable to access passion—not because you no longer want to feel passionate but because your biology has shut the door to that experience. Your energy is now solely focused on survival and passion is a luxury you can't afford.

From a state of regulation, you can connect with the strong and deep feelings that passion brings. Passion is a positive emotion that pulls you into investing time and energy in something that you do because of your love for it, not because you are paid to do it. It brings feelings of being in a flow, excitement, and deep satisfaction.

Discover what you are passionate about. Ask yourself:

- **What brings you great joy?**

- **What excites you?**

- **What do you love discovering more about?**

- **What do you want to spend time doing?**

While passion is something that nourishes you and brings a sense of well-being, purpose fills you by the ways you make a difference to others. It is what you feel called to bring to the world. Your sense of purpose may arise from challenges you've faced, or it may naturally develop over your lifetime. You may still be exploring what you are called to do or have found your purpose and are living it. Purpose brings meaning to life and like passion, from a state of survival, it is not possible. You are only able to focus on purpose when you feel safe and connected and are in a state of regulation.

To help you explore your purpose in life, ask yourself:

What do you feel called to do in the world?

What do you value most?

→ **What do you care about deeply?**

→ **What do you have to offer?**

→ **What are your skills and strengths?**

conclusion

We are works in progress, our autonomic nervous systems listening and learning in each moment. Tuning into the wisdom of the nervous system is an essential part of living a life of well-being and changes the way we see our own experiences and the way we see the world.

I like to think of daily life as an autonomic journey. Sometimes we struggle to keep our balance while other times we move easily through the day. Our nervous system is an embodied, biological resource that is always present and ready to guide us. The science tells us that with practice we can strengthen our connection to the biological state of safety and create new patterns of connection. We can learn to meet challenges with more equanimity and stop to celebrate the times when life feels more manageable. The nervous system knows the way to safety and connection—knows the way home to regulation—and is ready to help us get there.

Understanding how our autonomic nervous system works may take away the mystery of how we move through the world, but it also invites the magic of our human experience. When we understand how our biology creates the platform for our experiences and how our autonomic state sets the landscape for our stories, we can embrace the many magical moments that make life such an extraordinary, miraculous experience.

As we come to the end of the workbook, I hope you are on your way to finding the rhythm of regulation that brings you safety, connection, and joy. May you move through the day in a new way ready for an autonomic adventure . . . Deb

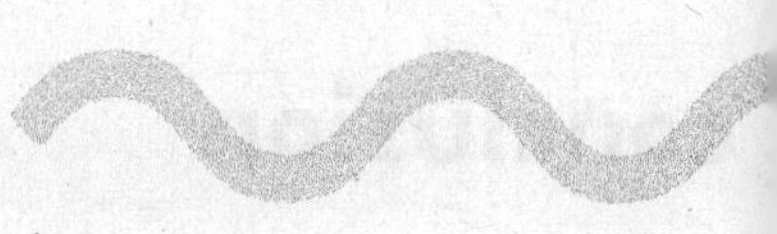

acknowledgments

Writing is a refuge for me. When I write, I escape the demands of daily life and enter the world of words. Every writing project has its own rhythm and brings different joys and challenges. This project brought a particular set of challenges. I began writing the workbook during the last year of my husband Bob's life and finished it after his death. Some days words flowed with ease and other days I struggled to put a single sentence together. Some days I reached for writing as a resource to make it through the day and other days writing was unthinkable. Bob was always a champion of my work, and I know it would bring him joy to see this book in its final form. The love and care of my family and friends continues to keep me going. My daughters have a special place in my heart, and my trusted group of friends remind me I'm not alone.

The Sounds True team were fantastic to work with. They had a vision for the workbook and partnered with me every step of the way. Writing a workbook was a new experience for me, and the team brought in a wonderful editor, Melissa Valentine, to help me find my workbook voice.

I'm deeply thankful for the work of my colleague and friend Stephen Porges. Without his development of Polyvagal Theory, our understanding of the nervous system would be incomplete, and we would not have the information needed to travel the pathways to well-being. An entire community of people helped me bring this work to life. I am holding each of you in my heart.

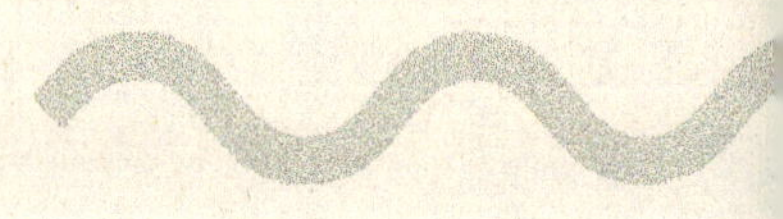

about the author

Deb Dana, LCSW, is a clinician and consultant specializing in using the lens of Polyvagal Theory to understand and resolve the impact of trauma and create ways of working that honor the role of the autonomic nervous system. She is a founding member of the Polyvagal Institute, clinical consultant to Khiron Clinics, and an advisor to Unyte. Deb's work shows how an understanding of Polyvagal Theory is applicable across the board to relationships, mental health, and trauma. She delves into the intricacies of how we can all use an understanding of the organizing principles of Polyvagal Theory to change the ways we navigate our daily lives. Deb is well known for translating Polyvagal Theory into a language and application that is both clear and accessible, and for pioneering Rhythm of Regulation® methodology, tools, techniques, and practices which continue to open up the power of Polyvagal Theory for professionals and curious people from diverse backgrounds and all walks of life.

Deb believes that we all benefit when we have a basic understanding of the ways the nervous system works and learn how to become active operators of this essential system. Following this passion has led her to offering workshops in partnership with groups and communities outside of the clinical arena—and bringing the Polyvagal perspective to the ordinary, and sometimes extraordinary, experiences of daily living.

Deb's publications include *Anchored: How to Befriend Your Nervous System Using Polyvagal Theory*, *The Polyvagal Theory in Therapy: Engaging the Rhythm of Regulation*, *Polyvagal Exercises for Safety and Connection: 50 Client-Centered Practices*, *Polyvagal Practices: Anchoring the Self in Safety*, *Polyvagal Prompts: Finding Connection and Joy Through Guided Explorations*, the *Polyvagal Card Deck*, the *Polyvagal Flip Chart*, and the audio program *Befriending Your Nervous System: Looking through the Lens of Polyvagal Theory*. To learn more, visit rhythmofregulation.com.